DEMENTIA,

YOU ARE NOT ALONE!

From the perspective of a former carer and now a person living with dementia

Michael Booth

Contents

Dedication i

About the Author ii

Foreword... 1

Scenario 2

    Explanation: 8

Background 10

Diagnosis Why and When?...................................14

Understanding your diagnosis and dementia as a whole 20

Young Onset Dementia.......................................27

Acceptance Coming to terms with your diagnosis. 34

Dealing with stigma..42

The value of family and a good support network 51

    Our dear valued carers.................................. 60

    If you have no family 63

Weighing up the positives and negatives for now and the future 66

Living Situation 73

    When to consider moving............................... 79

    Choosing a Suitable Home 81

    Care Home 86

Staying active physically and mentally.....................94

Volunteering. Why, how, when, and for whom?........ 103

Question & Answers 115

Why do people living with dementia get tired much quicker and sleep more? 116

As a carer, I am so tired, what can I do? 119

Can you feel the decline when you have dementia, and what does it feel like?......................................124

Why do a person's memories regress?.................127

Why do people living with dementia wander? 131

Should I lie to a person living with dementia? 134

Why does the person's behaviour change, and how can I handle that? 138

Conclusion 143

Acknowledgments.. 150

A special note to past, current, and early career researchers: 156

Dedication

I would like to dedicate this book to my family.

To my dear wife who put up with my nonsense whilst i was writing the book. You never complained once and helped me during the process. You are my wife, my best friend, and my rock.

Thank you so very much for being you.

About the Author

My experience with dementia started over 20 years ago. First, with my grandfather, who had late-stage dementia, though he refused to go to the doctor. My mom was diagnosed with Alzheimer's when she was around 56 years of age. Her symptoms started when she was in her early 50s.

Honestly, I knew nothing about dementia. Only that it was an older person's memory problem. An age thing. How wrong I was!

For secular work, I was a project manager and a business analyst. Dealing with quality, production, strategy, planning, training. My work, education, and curiosity has taught me that what I do not know or understand, I should research until I know enough to make a decision or plan ahead. This has served me well after my mom was diagnosed. I studied all types of dementia, which helped me understand as much as I could about the disease.

Little did I know that just a few months after my mom's death, I would be diagnosed as well with Alzheimer's at the age of 46.

I found that I was not the only one who knew very little about dementia, so I used what I learned to help and educate others. After my diagnosis, I found that the lack of support was just the same for me as it was for my mom when she was diagnosed 10 years earlier.

To my surprise though, I found that support is there. Unfortunately, you need to know where to look, and that led me to writing this book.

I hope what I have learned will help you, too.

Foreword

I will start by saying that I have no medical experience.

I have, however, done a lot of research and spoken to clinicians, people who care for someone with dementia, and those who have been diagnosed with dementia.

These are my thoughts, comments, and experiences. They are purely based on lived experience as a former carer for my mom, who was diagnosed with young onset dementia and my experience as a person now living with young onset dementia myself.

During the read you will see mentioned references to the Mental Health Services. This is what the mental health team are called in the area where I live. They will be available in your area but perhaps under a different name. If you ask your doctor or medical team for the mental health services that care for people living with dementia in your area, they will know what you mean, and they can point you in the right direction.

Scenario

I know something is wrong, but I am not sure what.

I cannot remember where I put my keys. I sometimes cannot remember where I am going. I go into a room and cannot remember why. I seem slower in comprehending things.

Nobody notices, and when they do, we can laugh it off. I mentioned these to my GP in passing. I was told it was most likely stress and that we will just monitor it.

As time moves on, I do not seem to be getting any better. In fact, some things are getting worse. I am struggling to find my words, I cannot keep up with conversations anymore, I ask or repeat the same things, I am not remembering appointments or to do things my family asks, my sleep is being disturbed, and I am starting to feel down. Whatever is going on is now starting to affect most things that I do.

I am trying hard to hide these issues, but most people are noticing, only now it is becoming a no laughing matter. Comments are made such as: "What is wrong with you?", "Stop being silly now!", "You're becoming irritating and no fun anymore." Even hurtful words have been overheard,

2

such as "stupid," "mad," "crazy," and "unbearable." I do not see my friends anymore; they think I am a bit weird.

My boss is starting to question my ability and ethic to work as I am not delivering on time, not remembering tasks assigned to me at meetings, or not even keeping up at meetings.

My children are noticing, too. The tranquillity of the house is being affected. More arguments ensue because I have not done something they asked me to, or I have forgotten something. They are getting fed up with me repeating things, forgetting things, or asking the same questions again and again. I do not blame them, really.

My relationship with my wife is suffering. It is like we are keeping apart more, living separate lives. The adage is true: *it's not you, it's me*. To keep the peace with my wife and children and to try and hide what I am going through, I am shutting myself off more and more.

I go to see my GP again and a short memory test is done: 3 simple things to remember and repeat back. Well, that did not go well! GP says it could be several things causing the issues but believes it is still stress and perhaps depression. Bloods are taken, and a low dose of an anti-depressant is prescribed. An appointment is to be made with a neurologist.

I get a letter that says my appointment to see the neurologist is going to be in 8 months' time, and that was followed by another letter moving the appointment back 4 months. I now must wait over a year to see the neurologist. I am struggling, and so are those around me. I cannot cope, I feel so alone, with no support.

I go back to the GP, and in broken, slow speech and tears, I explain that things are gradually getting worse. I can feel things are not right. I explain that my balance is off as well now. The GP increases my anti-depressant medication and says there is not much else they can do without consulting the Neurologist first.

I do not seem to speak to my friends anymore, not even a text or a call.

My boss has all but given me my last chance to improve, or they will have to replace me. I am not performing as well as I was, and I am off sick too often. I try to explain what I am going through, but it seems to fall on deaf ears.

One of my children is sympathetic to what I am going through and wants to help and support me through it. My other child says that she does not understand: I can remember some things but not others, so there cannot be anything wrong. She adds the comment that I am too young to be having problems like those I describe; those symptoms are for older people to have. She then adds that I should stop playing on some of the symptoms and making them worse by exaggerating things. She stays away from me.

My wife and I are constantly bickering and arguing. The home is just not a good place to be anymore. We are even speaking about separation and divorce.

It is breaking my heart to see the family that I love and cherish so dearly falling apart like this, and it seems to be all my fault. I feel so guilty, and no matter how hard I try, I seem powerless to change what I am going through or the effect it is having on others around me. I am heartbroken, alone and feeling useless.

I do eventually get to see the neurologist, and she orders an MRI scan; while I wait for that, I will do a cognitive and memory test.

I endured the cognitive and memory tests performed by a psychiatrist. It is hard, emotional, and embarrassing. I should know the answers to these questions, and I should be able to perform the tasks, but I cannot, and the result of the test is not good and way too young for my age.

I must wait another 4 months to see the neurologist again for any results, only to be told the results of the MRI are inconclusive. A more in-depth scan called a SPECT scan is to be ordered.

I am barely holding it together at this point and I am only just keeping my family together with my fingernails. The feelings of uselessness, guilt, and being alone are becoming overwhelming. We are almost 4 years on from when I first spoke to the GP, and yet we are no further forward.

Getting the SPECT scan was stressful. Being strapped in and told not to move a muscle for 10 minutes was hard. I had to do it twice because, guess what, I moved something but cannot remember what.

I did a 2nd cognitive and memory test with the psychiatrist, and the score was worse than the first time. I also get to see the neurologist again for my scan results.

The diagnosis is not good. The full neurological report shows that despite my age, I have a form of dementia called young-onset Alzheimer's.

The neurologist tells me that because of my age and the stage that the Alzheimer's is at, I can try the medication that slows the progression. She also tells me that there is nothing else they can do for me and hands me a handful of leaflets on things I should consider regarding my future.

My partner and I cry; she apologises for not believing me. My boss is not so forgiving - he says that due to the diagnosis, I cannot work there as it's too much of a risk. He terminates my employment on the grounds of ill health.

My own daughter still cannot accept this and says I am too young. My friends, I never hear from anymore.

Despite my diagnosis, the feelings of being alone, guilty, and useless just do not go away.

I lose my driver's licence as well as my job. We go from 2 healthy salaries to now just 1 in a matter of a week after my diagnosis. Everything has fallen apart after a very tiring 4-year battle to get a diagnosis.

What do I do now?

Explanation:

The scenario has been made up of my experience with my mom, some of the things I have been through, and some added details from the experiences of others in the Young Onset Dementia group I belong to

Many have expressed to me that their experiences echo that of mine. How sad this is.

The scenario describes the breaking down of families and how partners and children walk out on the person living with dementia. It was heart-wrenching to listen as some told me their experiences - sadly, this is all too common and generally because the diagnosis process takes too long and because of the stigma attached to dementia and the uncertainty of the future for everyone affected.

The feeling of guilt, uselessness and being alone was a common thread for us all, including myself. We have all dealt with this differently and in our own ways.

What you are going to read is how I have dealt with things moving forward and how I helped my dad care for my mom.

I hope that this will help you whether you are diagnosed, a carer, someone going through the diagnostic process, or simply wanting to learn and understand dementia better.

If you are afraid to get a diagnosis for whatever reason, I hope it motivates you to do so and not to be afraid of getting diagnosed or the stigma attached to dementia.

If you are a carer, I hope to help you care for your loved one the best way you can.

Whatever your situation,

YOU ARE NOT ALONE!

Background

My lived experience with dementia started in 2005 when my mom showed signs of cognitive impairment. It took a frustratingly painful four years before she was diagnosed as having Alzheimer's with aphasia (known as Lopogenic Progressive Aphasia). At the time of her diagnosis, my mom was just 56 years of age.

Caring for somebody who is diagnosed with dementia can be, let us say, challenging at the best of times, especially as the disease progresses, but add aphasia to the mix, and it becomes even more challenging. Knowing what my mom needed and when she needed it was difficult at the best of times. My mom passed away at the age of 66 in a care home. The decision of when to move her into a care home was a very long and difficult process as there were many factors to consider, including separating my dad and mum, who'd been married for nearly 50 years.

The neurologist investigated everything except dementia simply because of her age at the time. By the time she was diagnosed, it was too far advanced, and the medication that could have slowed it down would have served no purpose for her. The neurologist said sympathetically that it was dementia, specifically Alzheimer's and that there was nothing they could do for her. Then, they handed my dad a load of leaflets to read and discharged her from their services. That was it. No guidance, no direction on what to do next, no follow-up, and nothing about the disease.

The leaflets dealt with getting things such as legal power of attorney, wills, and care homes for later-stage dementia. Sound advice, as we will discuss later, but nothing that would be of any help straight after being told you have a degenerative disease that will take your life.

I was diagnosed with Alzheimer's disease at the age of 47. This disease affects all 4 quadrants of my brain from an early stage, not just memory. My balance and visual and spatial awareness are affected, which results in falls. Any unevenness in the floor, changing floor colour or texture can result in me being unbalanced. Going up and down stairs is incredibly challenging. In just three years, I visited A&E four times for various breaks and fractures because of falls. Driving, planning a journey or even knowing where I am at times is a problem for me.

The diagnosis process you read in the "Scenario" was my journey only. I used the mental health team and then the neurologist to later confirm the diagnosis, as you will read later.

10 years after my mom was diagnosed, I was handed the exact same leaflet. Nothing in 10 years had changed on the diagnosis front!

The scenario also mentions the loss of my driver's license, my work and going from 2 salaries down to 1 in just one week. That is also true.

My wife was very supportive through the whole process and still is today. I do not have two children, only one, my precious son.

By doing a lot of research for my dad and I on the disease, we were able to care for my mom the best we could. There is useful information out there - you just need to know where to look. Saying that, there is also quite a bit of rubbish or misinformation out there as well. On top of that, there are gaps in the information you may need; for example, there is not much information available that really guides you into when is the best time to move or even where to move to. Should I move into a care home, or should I move into supported living?

Without the correct advice and information, it is difficult to know what to do, when, and how to do it. So, I would like to talk you through the process I went through to firstly find the support I needed, and then, secondly, using that support to try and help me and my dad, and later me and my wife, make decisions, adaptions, plans and understanding of what is happening. This, I hope will help either yourself or your loved one.

The aim, really, is to help you, as a diagnosed person, live with the disease the best you can, and if you are caring, to care for your loved one in the best way you can use my lived experience coupled with research and useful advice that was given to me.

At the end of each section, I have left space for you to make your own notes on your thoughts and action plans you would like, or need to take, now, or in the future.

Diagnosis
Why and When?

Based on what I have just said about what happened with my mom and her diagnosis process, which, sad to say, is quite normal for the diagnosis process, there does not seem to be much purpose in getting diagnosed with a dementia. But I would recommend that you do. Why?

Let me tell you about my diagnosis first. My diagnosis process was very different from that of my mom's, but that's only because of a very astute mental health team that was helping with the care of my mom, who was alert to what I was going through. Let me explain.

During the later stage of my mum's dementia path, she was admitted into a mental health hospital where they care for people with organic health issues. In my mom's case, it was her aggressive or violent outbreaks and her neither eating nor drinking that was of major concern, and so they admitted her.

(From a clinical point of view, mental health issues are broken up into two categories. The first is functional. Things such as Autism, ADHD, clinical depression, etc, fall into this category. The second is organic. Dementia and other brain-related degenerative diseases fall in this category.)

While speaking to the psychologist and the mental health team about my mom's palliative care, she noted that I was repeating certain questions and not following some of the conversation. At the end of the meeting, she pulled me aside and asked how I was doing; she explained what she had noted. I said it was probably just because I was stressed about what was happening with my mum and how my dad was handling it. It was a stressful time!

Dementia was truly the last thing I was thinking about for myself. I lived healthy. Never smoked, hardly drank alcohol, and had an active lifestyle.

Nonetheless, she advised that there would be no harm in taking the memory cognitive test. I did that test and scored very low for my age. (This was perhaps the most humiliating thing I have ever done. I couldn't answer questions that I should have known. Things I should have been able to remember or identify, I couldn't. It was tiring and, as I said, humiliating.)

A full family history was done, as well as a description of other symptoms that I was dealing with. After this was done, everything was then double-checked separately with my wife in case I had omitted anything. Honestly, it felt like they were double-checking everything to see that I was telling the truth. It felt like an interrogation. However, it is not that way at all. The clinicians simply need all the facts from you and those closest to you. Let's face it: we can cover up what is really happening, or we can exaggerate. They need the facts to investigate fully, so please try to be a bit humble here and allow the clinicians to do their job properly.

This investigation led to scans being ordered. A full neuro workup was carried out with a few different types of scans. All the investigatory work done led to a diagnosis of Alzheimer's disease. The diagnosis process for me, due to the alertness of the mental health team and the psychologist, only took just over a year, which shows that it can be done quicker if the clinicians and general practitioners are alert to the fact that this could be dementia!

As a result of an early diagnosis, I was able to get the medication that slows the disease down.

Now, there is a lot of debate currently in the scientific research community as to whether the medication helps at all. All I can say is that I was struggling with my speech and memory was worse before I got the medication, but after a few months of taking the medication, my speech started to improve, and so did my memory, to the point that I can now do public speaking again. I will leave it to you to debate whether the medication works or not. From my point of view, I felt it helped me. How long will the medication work for? That, I do not know.

Your doctor may not refer you to the mental health services but rather to a neurologist. If you take the neurologist route, it will take longer to get a diagnosis simply because there are not enough neurologists in this country; thus, the waiting time is long. I suggest insisting with your doctor to go to the mental health services from the very beginning. I asked to do both. Make an appointment with the mental health team as well as the neurologist. My thinking was that the mental health team are qualified and specialised in dementia diagnosis. They can do a full neuro workup (including asking the doctor to book scans). You will most likely have the diagnosis before you get to see a neurologist! I simply used the neurologist to get a second opinion and to double-check the diagnosis. That is just me, though. If you want to rule dementia out or get a diagnosis, then the mental health team is the quickest route, in my opinion. You will also get better support during the process.

So, taking the length of time, it might take to get a diagnosis, some of the humiliating questions that are done in the cognitive test, and whether the medication works or not, and accepting that there is currently no cure for dementia, why get diagnosed because it all seems rather negative?

This is my reasoning:

Going through all the above and getting a diagnosis is important! Why?

Medication, support, planning, and understanding for yourself and others.

Not knowing leaves things up in the air and people wondering what is wrong with you. In some cases, some, which could include your own family members, think you are fooling around or playing on symptoms.

Once diagnosed, support can come in many ways, as we will discuss, but that support is only there *if* you get diagnosed!

Key Points:

Get a Diagnosis.

Getting a diagnosis answers a lot of questions and doubts.

The diagnostic process is hard to do and takes a while, but do not let that put you off.

The benefits of a diagnosis far out way the negatives when it comes to support and medication.

You can do everything correct in your life and still be at risk of getting dementia due to genetics.

YOUR NOTES AND THOUGHTS:

Understanding your diagnosis and dementia as a whole

What is dementia?

"The word dementia derives from the Latin root 'demens', which means being out of one's mind. Although the term "dementia" has been used since the 13th century, its mention in the medical community was reported in the 18th century". - National Library of Medicine, United States of America- History of dementia - 2018

Other words used historically are "senile", "crazy", and "confused". Because of such connotations, some object to the use of the word dementia, preferring instead the term "Multi Neurocognitive Disease" (MND).

I recognise their efforts to have the term dementia changed, but I will continue to use this term simply because that is what most people know the disease as.

"Dementia is a group of symptoms that is caused by different diseases that damage the brain. Dementia is progressive, which means symptoms may be relatively mild at first, but they get worse over time. There are many types of dementia, but Alzheimer's disease is the most common. The next most common is vascular dementia.

Dementia is not a natural part of ageing. It is caused when a disease damages nerve cells in the brain. Nerve cells carry messages between different parts of the brain and to other parts of the body. As more nerve cells are damaged, the brain becomes less able to work properly. Dementia can be caused by many different diseases. These diseases affect the brain in different ways, resulting in different types of dementia." – Alzheimer's Society 2023 - www.alzheimers.org.uk/about-dementia/types-dementia/what-is-dementia

So, put simply, dementia is an umbrella term for different types of diseases that cause the brain to degenerate over time. In much the same way, cancer is an umbrella term for different types of cancers that effect different areas of the body. Unlike a lot of cancers though these days, dementia has no cure and is thus a terminal disease.

There are an estimated 100 types of dementia. These include Alzheimer's, Vascular dementia, Lewd body, Frontal Temporal dementia (formally known as Picks disease), as well as things such as Creutzfeldt-Jakob disease, Wernicke-Korsakoff's dementia, Parkinson's disease, and Huntington's disease. The most common form is Alzheimer's, with 60 to 70% of diagnosed persons having this type of dementia.

Some will argue that dementia does not kill you, that something else will cause your death, not the dementia, and yet I have just called it a terminal disease. Why?

I will reason on it this way. Does cancer kill?

You will most likely say yes if untreated cancer will cause your death. You would be correct! However, most times, it is a weak immune system that will cause a virus or infection that will take your life, not so much the cancer. In realistic terms, it would be complications due to cancer. Despite this, we accept today that cancer kills.

The same is true with all types of dementia. We will most likely die from complications due to dementia, so therefore, dementia, like cancer, kills.

Think about it: the brain controls everything, including our eating, drinking, and breathing. As the brain degenerates, we stop eating and drinking, and eventually, the brain cannot send the signals for our heart to pump, and we stop breathing.

Compare your brain to a computer or a mobile phone. They are controlled by hardware that causes the device to work the way it should, the way it is intended to operate. But if that piece of hardware were to get corrupted in some way, perhaps by a virus, the computer or phone would stop working correctly. If we left the device and did nothing, over time, the device would stop working. It would die!

Dementia is the same. For reasons not fully understood yet, our brains stop working correctly. It gets worse over time, working less and less until the brain shrinks to the point where it stops working.

Dementia kills! So do not let anyone tell you otherwise. Ignorance is no longer bliss...

An especially important note here!

When getting a diagnosis, get to know not just the type but also the *subtype* of dementia that you have. Why is that important?

The type and subtype of your dementia can identify both the speed and the aggressiveness of the disease.

It is believed that there are over 200 subtypes of dementia. As an example, let us consider the more common Alzheimer's disease. In its simplest form, Alzheimer's disease can be divided into typically 2 subtypes. There is Amnesiac Alzheimer's disease, where the damage first appears in the hippocampus - this is the most typical of the Alzheimer's disease. Then there is the Atypical Alzheimer's disease, which can be subtyped into three areas: Posterior Cortical Atrophy [PCA], Lopogenic Progressive Aphasia [LPA], and Dysexecutive Alzheimer's Disease [DAD]. (There are other subtypes but for the sake of simplicity, I have just mentioned the most common.)

Each one of these subtypes acts differently and can be found in various parts of the brain. PCA, for example, affects the Occipital Lobes and the Parietal Lobes. This means that in the early stages, memory may not be affected; things such as spatial awareness, visual impairment, hearing, and balance will be affected more. I have read that, in some cases, people with PCA can see things upside down as though they are walking on the ceiling.

LPA causes damage to the left side of the Temporal Lobe and the Parietal Lobe. This means early signs would be those affecting speech, such as not being able to find the right words to say in a conversation or not following conversations.

DAD affects the Frontal Lobes of the brain. Early symptoms would include difficulties with planning, organising, initiation, judgement, and the ability to make decisions.

Each one of these types and subtypes progresses differently and affects people differently.

As the disease progresses, though, they all merge into one, commonly known as Late-Stage Dementia. But knowing the type of dementia that you have early on and the subtype will mean that you will know what type of journey you are going to have, how that subtype will affect you, and what planning and support might be needed.

Dementia is different for each person, and so the future can look different for each person. Based on the experience of others previously diagnosed, my own experience of watching my mom go through her journey, and my own lived experience leads me to believe what my future will be like. My subtype is a mixed Alzheimer's, as the disease affects all 4 quadrants of the brain. What I do not know is how long that journey will take.

Despite not knowing how long it will take for this disease to take everything I have; I can still prepare now for that day.

For more information on the type of dementia diagnosed, I suggest researching your specific type.

Key Points:

Try not to get too hung up on the word 'dementia'. It is the medically accepted term all over the world. It may, in time, change.

Know not just the type of dementia you have but also the subtype. This will help you to prepare for the future.

YOUR NOTES AND THOUGHTS:

Young Onset Dementia

Young Onset Dementia is not a type of dementia. It is a description of someone who has been diagnosed with a type of dementia at a younger age.

"Dementia is described as 'young onset' when symptoms develop before the age of 65, usually between 30 to 65 years of age. It is also referred to as 'early onset' or 'working age' dementia, but these terms can cause confusion. 'Early onset' can be interpreted as the early stages of dementia and is applicable to people of any age and 'working age' is now less defined as retirement age is more flexible.

There are differences in the types of dementia commonly diagnosed in younger people compared to those of an older age. For example, only about a third of dementia diagnosed in younger people are of the Alzheimer's type in comparison to about 60% in the older age group." - Dementia UK 2023 - www.dementiauk.org/information-and-support/young-onset-dementia/what-is-young-onset-dementia/

Age makes it hard for a younger person to adjust to a diagnosis. Dementia can also be harder for younger people because it usually comes at a time in their life when it is least expected.

What is the difference between young-onset dementia and dementia in older persons?

Younger people (under the age of 65) affected by dementia are more likely to have the following issues which affect them differently than older persons, such as:

Have a rarer form of dementia affecting behaviour and social functioning.

There could be a genetic form of dementia, such as in my case. This creates an issue with my son as well. Does he get tested or not?

They will most likely experience employment issues, which could result in significant financial difficulties (such as struggling to pay a mortgage when they go from 2 salaries down to 1).

They could have children that are dependants or caring for elderly parents or relatives. All of the above significantly increases the chance of psychological and physical distress, as well as dealing with the challenges dementia brings.

"Children can find it difficult to come to terms with a parent having dementia. The person with dementia may feel guilty about the impact their diagnosis has on their

children. It can also affect the relationships between other members of the family. There can be difficulties balancing the needs of the person with dementia, their children and other family members. For example, it can be a challenge to support children emotionally and help them cope with the changes in a parent. It can be particularly hard for the parent without dementia or other family members who will need to provide more support for the family while also trying to meet the needs of the person with dementia".

Alzheimer's Society 2024 - www.alzheimers.org.uk/about-dementia/types-dementia/particular-issues-faced-younger-people-dementia

Some of these challenges might include one, some, or all of these symptoms:

Personality, behaviour, and language which leads to a social functioning challenge.

Relationships with others will become a problem, be that with family or friends, as the person could become withdrawn.

Activities of everyday living suffer due to a lack of motivation, concentration levels, mood, and depression. Decision-making and solving issues become a challenge, promoting frustration and sometimes anger.

Physical challenges such as vision, spatial awareness, balance, and motor skills become affected.

The challenges faced by a person with young onset, such as myself, can lead to them feeling useless (as mentioned in the scenario). That was certainly how I felt, and I was not alone - others told me the same thing when I spoke to them.

"After their diagnosis, younger people with dementia and their families may find that friends and other family members do not stay in touch or provide the support they need. This can be for different reasons. Dementia in a younger person is unexpected, so friends and family may not understand what the person and those close to them are going through". – Alzheimer's Society 2024 - www.alzheimers.org.uk/about-dementia/types-dementia/particular-issues-faced-younger-people-dementia

As you will see when you read on, the support for young onset is not always available, simply because of my age. Tell me, where is the fairness in that?

Despite my age and my diagnosis, it is still possible to learn new things, to get on with life and enjoy my time with my family. It just takes a little planning and forethought.

I must admit, it is not easy dealing with dementia at a younger age, knowing that it is only going to get worse as time goes on. If it was not for the support of my family and some very good friends I have made along the way, I am not sure how I would cope or even if I would want to cope.

I struggle with not being able to work anymore. Yes, I just said that! Seeing my wife work fulltime so that we can pay the bills and then care for me is hard to see and cope with. She is my rock!

I hope you have that rock as well, someone who does not mind the rants or the crying on the shoulder as you try to deal with the diagnosis. Someone who does not retaliate when you go through your mood swings. You will need that person for support.

Isolating yourself is never the answer, as much as you want to climb in that hole and never come out. Use your emotions to build up that all-important support network.

In case you are wondering, did my son get tested or not?

We discussed all the facts that we could find, and I spoke to a few specialists that I have encountered. Together, we then looked at the positives and negatives of knowing or not knowing. He is currently 25 years old at the time of writing this.

After a discussion of the facts, we left the decision up to him. His decision was, for now, not to get tested. His reasoning was that he wants to live his life without the additional stress and if it happens, it happens, and we will deal with it then.

That was his choice. You may choose differently, and that is ok too.

My brother, who is 8 years younger than me (42), has already started to show signs of cognitive decline and has been diagnosed with MCI (mild cognitive impairment).

This is very difficult for my dad to deal with. He has just seen my mom live through and pass away from a terrible disease, and now he has one son diagnosed with dementia and another with MCI. I feel for him. But we are here for him despite our challenges.

This disease is never easy, no matter your age. Acceptance will be one of the hardest things that I think you will ever have to deal with. It certainly was for me and many others that I spoke to. But it can be done, how?

Key point:

Young Onset Dementia will come with more challenges simply because of the age at which the person is diagnosed. The earlier the diagnosis, the worse it will be.

More support will be required in areas not normally thought of when diagnosed with dementia.

YOUR NOTES AND THOUGHTS:

Acceptance

Coming to terms with your diagnosis.

Getting a diagnosis of any type of dementia is extremely hard and sometimes can be difficult to accept, whether you are the person being diagnosed or a person who will now take on the role of their carer. It can be like a heavy blow to the gut!

Time and patience are needed to digest the diagnosis that you have just been given. These two attributes will be your new buzz words while you are on the journey to acceptance, but during this period, if possible, try to avoid making any major decisions. Making a major decision during this period could result in a decision that you may come to regret or that may make it harder for you or your carer to accept the diagnosis.

So, step one is to emotionally deal with your diagnosis to the point of acceptance.

What do I mean by acceptance?

Acceptance does not mean that you stop living or that there is nothing that you can do about your diagnosis. Acceptance simply means coming to terms with your

34

diagnosis and the limitations that this may place on you. Acceptance also implies learning to adapt to your new situation, even in the smallest of ways, which will be of immense help.

To do this, you will need support - support from your loved ones who will also be struggling to come to terms with the diagnosis (and so patience will be needed from everyone by everyone), support from medical clinicians, support from various charities, even support from technology (I found Alexa and a digital calendar helpful). Make use of these to the best of your ability. Insist on the support that you need, and sadly, it is a matter of *insisting* on what you need when it comes to dementia. I found it useful speaking to a psychologist to help me deal with my emotions, bearing in mind I just lost my mom to the same disease. I realised that this is not to everyone's liking but I do recommend it or at least speaking to someone that you can trust and that will not judge how you're feeling.

Everything will run through your head. From "What will my future look like?" and "Will my loved ones manage to care for me and what effect it will have on them?" to "Will I be able to do certain things?" and "What about my ability to care for myself and my independence?" You will think back to the things you once could do without even thinking about it but can now no longer do either with ease or at all.

All these thoughts, though natural and certainly not wrong, are frustrating, to say the least, and to linger on them is not good for your emotional or mental state.

Emotions will run high; tempers can flare; words can be said that are not meant in the heat of the moment. Speaking to someone can alleviate or, at the very least, help you to deal with these emotions.

Perhaps a word of caution here:

Try not to use a loved one close to you as the person you choose to open-up to about your emotions. This is because they are most likely feeling the same, if not similar, emotions. Knowing how you are struggling can make it harder for them to come to terms with the diagnosis. They will generally try to help you deal with these emotions at the expense of their own. Sometimes, all you need is someone to listen to you and to help you work through your questions and concerns yourself.

A wise and trusted friend gave me an illustration to help me cope with my thoughts and emotions.

You only have two legs, but there are three circles. The first circle is your past, the 2nd circle is your present, and the 3rd circle is your future. With both of your legs together, you will stand in the 2nd circle, in the present. When you think about the past it is quite easy, due to the emotions that you face as you think about things you once could do and now struggle with, to move both feet into the first circle, your past, and get stuck there. This can prevent you from living in the present! The opposite is also true, where you could move both feet into the future, the 3rd circle. The problem here is that you think about all the things that will go wrong and the future that dementia will bring to you. Again, you miss the present!

How can we move to the past or to the future, in that we step into circles one or three but still live in the present without allowing the emotions, the anxieties, and perhaps even depression to stop us from living now?

By keeping one foot always in the 2nd circle! Always keep one foot in the present.

There's nothing wrong with stepping back in time and thinking what you could once do and, from that learn to adapt. There's also nothing wrong with stepping into the future, thinking about what could occur and making plans.

But by keeping one foot firmly planted in the 2nd circle, in the present, we will always come back to the present. By doing this we help to keep our emotions and anxieties in check. Doing this will take a bit of practice and, again, support.

Once you feel ready, and that you have accepted the diagnosis, you can look to make a decision that will suit both you and your family. At that time, speak openly to all those concerned about the struggles you may be having, for example, in your own home, or if you have concern for one of your loved ones and the situation they face in their own home, try to openly discuss this with them.

I use the home situation as an example simply because this is a noticeably big decision (and one we will discuss later), but it could be anything that you need support with.

I will be honest here, what I have just said may make it sound like it's easy to accept the diagnosis. It really is not easy! In fact, many people never come to terms with their diagnosis, and a family member may never accept that their father or mother has dementia, which can cause major splits in a family. Some family members who are dear to the person diagnosed simply walk away and never have anything to do with their loved one again. Please, do not be that person. Whether you accept the diagnosis or not, your father, mother, brother, sister, son, daughter, or friend needs you now more than ever, and your support will mean the world to them (even though they may not say so).

If you are the person diagnosed and you do not want to accept your diagnosis or find it hard to accept, this will, over time, only cause you and your family frustrations (which will most probably cause you to drive your loved ones away). They can only do so much to support you, but if you do not allow them to do so, what can they do? Argue or fight with you? Many will, and resentment can set in.

My advice to you is to try your best to accept the diagnosis or, at the very least, accept that you need support. Your loved ones will always be discreet - they love you, and they want the best for you, for you to be comfortable. Allow them to do so. Be open with them and keep the lines of communication open. Let them know you need some support and what support, or how much support, you need. You may need no help at all. Let them know, 'you got this!'

You do not want to be alone when you need support the most. I have seen that, and it is not pretty.

If you are alone and have no family, dementia will be the hardest thing you will ever have to deal with. You will need to still live and all that that entails, but to do so alone will be extremely hard. If you can, speak to your closest of friends and explain what is going on and what your future looks like. Ask them to be that friend that will support you. The more the merrier!

If you do not have those close friends. Contact your social worker or the Admiral nurses for advice.

For myself, due to the falls that I was having and the very real reality that soon I would do some serious damage to myself, I had an open discussion with my wife and explained the problems and issues that I was facing in the house. We looked at trying to make modifications in the house, but this was going to be very costly. Also, because I was diagnosed with dementia and not able to work anymore, this created a financial strain on top of all the other issues we have just discussed. I was able to do some modifications myself, but it still was not enough. My wife was very supportive in providing what I needed. It was incredibly sad to have to discuss and then come to the realisation, that perhaps it was time to move.

We will discuss this in more detail a bit later on.

Key Points:

Take time to digest your diagnosis and avoid making heavy decisions during this time.

Seek support and advice, someone that you can openly talk too. I suggest, based on my experience not a close family member but, if you can, a professional.

Consider everyone's emotions, we are *all* having to deal with the diagnosis.

Stay in the present.

Be open and honest about the concerns you have.

Get the help and support you need; this will help you accept the diagnosis.

YOUR NOTES AND THOUGHTS:

Dealing with stigma

Part of accepting the diagnosis is to deal with stigma.

Stigma is based on bias and stereotypes - quite often unconscious bias that we all have in one form or another.

Stigma - "a mark of disgrace associated with a particular circumstance, quality, or person" – *Online Oxford Dictionary 2023*

Some work that was done by the Bradford university in conjunction with people living with young onset dementia, including myself, came up with this explanation on stigma and stereotypes.

As a side note - I would like to add what a great pleasure and an honour to work with Bradford University – Centre for Applied Dementia Studies and those living with dementia to develop, publish, and teach the very first MSc in dementia studies developed with people living with came up with this explanation on stigma and stereotypes.

Collectively, we came up with this explanation on stigma and stereotypes:

"Unconscious bias refers to the automatic and unintentional biases or prejudices that individuals hold towards certain groups of people, based on various

characteristics such as race, gender, age, disability, appearance, or socioeconomic status. These biases are formed and operate at a subconscious level, outside of our awareness and control, influencing our attitudes, beliefs, and behaviours towards others.

Unconscious biases are rooted in social conditioning, cultural influences, and personal experiences. They are a natural part of human cognition and can affect how we perceive, judge, and interact with individuals or groups, often leading to discriminatory or unfair treatment, even when we consciously believe in equality and fairness.

Research has shown that unconscious biases can significantly impact various aspects of life. These biases often support negative stereotypes that reinforce inequality.

It is important to note that unconscious biases are not indicative of a person's character or intentions. They are deeply ingrained and often operate outside of our conscious awareness, meaning we may not be aware that we hold them.

Stereotypes and unconscious bias are closely related concepts. While they are distinct, they often intersect and reinforce each other.

Stereotypes are generalised beliefs or assumptions about a particular group of people. They are often oversimplified and may not reflect the true diversity and individuality. Stereotypes can be based on race, gender, age, religion, ethnicity, nationality, disability, or any other characteristic. They are deeply ingrained in society and can shape our perceptions, expectations, and interactions with individuals belonging to those groups.

Unconscious biases often draw from and reinforce stereotypes. As we grow up in a society that is saturated with stereotypes, they become deeply embedded in our subconscious minds. These stereotypes can shape our automatic associations and responses towards different people, leading to biased judgments, decisions, and discrimination.

"Women can't drive", "Blondes are dumb", and "men can't cook" – these are all common stereotypes.

Understanding what stereotypes are and how they influence our unconscious as well as conscious thoughts and actions is important for identifying how to overcome these and, furthermore, how to change the stigma and discrimination that often results.

Like many other disabilities, dementia is subject to stereotyping. The common assumptions made about people who live with dementia as a group are that they "are victims suffering from a disease", that "they cannot learn new things", and "they can't make decisions for themselves".

Stereotypes are often formed by the way dementia is represented by the news media and in popular culture. In recent years, there have been several characters with dementia in radio and TV soaps and drama series. These sources are often more interested in creating dramatic effects than in giving an authentic representation of dementia, and this is particularly true of the timescale over which dementia is typically shown to develop.

Dementia is often overwhelmingly associated with cognitive decline and memory loss. This association can lead to the perception that individuals with dementia are no longer capable, competent, or valuable members of society. Such stereotypes can undermine the personhood of people living with dementia.

Efforts to reduce dementia stigma have gained momentum in recent years, with campaigns focused on raising awareness, challenging stereotypes, and promoting dementia-friendly practices. The focus has shifted towards emphasising the personhood of individuals with dementia, highlighting their abilities, and encouraging supportive and inclusive communities.

While progress has been made in recent decades, dementia stigma and misconceptions still exist in many societies.

Results from an online survey in 2012 showed that 75% of people with dementia experienced negative association, and 40% reported being treated negatively, including losing friends and being isolated. Approximately one in four people with dementia still attempt to conceal their diagnosis from others due to the stigma associated with the disease. Alzheimer's Disease International (ADI) (2012) World Alzheimer's Report: Overcoming the Stigma of dementia. Available at https://www.alzint.org/resource/world-alzheimer-report-2012/

Ongoing efforts are needed to continue challenging these negative attitudes, promoting understanding, and providing support to individuals and families affected by dementia". - Taken from Centre for Applied Dementia Studies, Bradford University (2023) Understanding the me in dementia module study guide.

People generally think of late-stage dementia when you mention that you are diagnosed or they hear you have it, which makes the stigma for young onset dementia even worse. Not only do you have to deal with the normal stigma linked to dementia, but you will also have to deal with the added stigma of being too young, not being able to work, cannot manage your finances, and speak for yourself.

Some will say they do not notice anything different like your head is supposed to fall off or something. On a good day, that may well be the case, it may be that I am able to function fairly normally, but they don't often get to see behind closed doors.

How can you deal with stigma?

Is stigma preventing you from getting a diagnosis or preventing you from telling your family about your diagnosis?

If you allow it, stigma can begin to define who you are as a person. It can overtake you, and you start to believe what people say (like what was said to some in the scenario).

Stigma does not have to define you!

How you deal with stigma will come down to how you view yourself and the disease. The disease is not you. The disease is part of you, and we cannot get away from that, but we are not our disease! I will try to be me for as long as I possibly can.

That is the way I view and deal with stigma. I use the opportunity to educate and correct, politely of course. As we have said, the stigma is because of what they have been told or read in the past. Time moves on and, so re-educating people is the best way I have found to deal with this.

Some are just ignorant, and I just walk away from those – "horse to water" comes to mind. My life is complicated and frustrating enough living with this disease without having to deal with those people. Pick your battles.

I can just switch off and ignore some things even though they are wrong. If I feel the time is not right or it may be embarrassing for them, such as if we are in a meeting or group; I would rather speak to them in a quiet and private place. Others cannot do this and fly off the handle like a hammer to a nail. I have never seen that end well.

My suggestion is to be patient, bide your time, pick your battles, and remember to be polite. We want them to go away feeling educated, not browbeaten, because that way they will educate others as well.

By doing this, not only will it help you to deal with this annoying stigma, but you can play your part in rectifying that stigma.

The more people we have around us who are educated, the easier it becomes for you when it comes to support and guidance.

It is challenging telling your family about the diagnosis. Be open and honest about the diagnosis and how you feel. Allow them time to digest what you have just told them, and be prepared to answer questions. Their questions and responses will most likely be based on stigma. Help and guide them with love so that they can get an understanding of how you feel and what you need from them. It may be nothing right now, but you most certainly will need them later, so it is best to help them understand patiently.

After saying all the above, remember, never let stigma define you or stop you from getting a diagnosis. Stigma, as irritating and as ignorant as it is, is nothing to fear – you can handle stigma!

Key Points:

Dealing with stigma and stereotypes is not easy, but it can be done.

Pick your battles. You don't need to fight everything and all at once.

Be patient with everyone and treat people how you would like to be treated.

YOUR NOTES AND THOUGHTS:

The value of family and a good support network

I know I've mentioned it previously about considering others and the required support that you may need, but let's discuss in a little more detail what is available, where you will struggle to find suitable support, and how, if you let them, your family can be a great support to you.

I have referred to support, help, and assistance a few times now and will refer to it more as you read on, but what do I mean by support?

When some think about the word support, they think about someone holding their arm and helping them across the road or upstairs. Though this will be the case as the dementia progresses, it is not necessarily what I am referring to in each case.

Support can come in various ways. It may well be physical support you require, but it could also be emotional, psychological, financial, caring, or even all the above.

Whatever support you need or think you may need in the future, it is good to get it as early as possible. Building up a good network for support will serve you well when you need it the most.

That is easier said than done!

Building up a support network is not easy to do, especially when you require that support now or you're dealing with a new diagnosis. Nonetheless, it is well worth the effort. How do you go about getting a good support network?

As we have mentioned before, dementia does not just affect the person diagnosed. It affects all of those around them. This includes the emotions that you go through. When you are diagnosed with dementia, it can often feel like the end, that there is no hope, and that soon all you will be doing is sitting in your chair with a blank face. Honestly, this could not be further from the truth!

You will, however, face some challenging emotions. Feeling down or depressed, anger, frustration, sometimes self-loathing. Many questions will run through your head: What could I have done differently to avoid this? Why me? What will my future look like? How will my loved ones react? Will they care for me later? These are just some of the questions that went through my head.

Do not feel bad about these questions, it is a natural process very similar to the grieving process. Give yourself time to deal with these, and if needed, again, I will stress - seek support.

Start by talking about your dementia to your friends and family. Not all the time, as you do not want to chase them away. You know what I mean? Don't be that irritating person who cannot speak about anything else, but rather do so as you need too. You will most likely find that they know someone who is going through something similar, and they may be able to find out what they do or who supports them.

Bear in mind, too, though, that you will not be the only one going through these emotions or who has these questions. Your closest family members, your dearest loved ones, will be going through the same emotions and asking the same questions - all too often, though they bottle these up. Sad to say, many are not open about their emotions. Whether you are the diagnosed person or the loved one, we generally don't talk about dementia and the feelings and questions that are associated with it. My advice? Do not be like that! Openly speak to each other, let each other know how you feel, what questions you have, and the answers that you seek. By being open with each other, you all get the best support network possible, and where you cannot support each other or still find it a struggle, seek assistance and advice.

You might also find that when you research your type of dementia, you may come across a support group. This may not be local but rather online; it's still worth contacting them, though, to start building up that network (whether you need the support now or not). If you want local support, speak to the mental health team; maybe they will be able to direct you to a support group you can go to in person.

There are many places you can go to get advice and support, though sadly, they are not always openly advertised. The NHS, for example, will have a mental health team in your area. To get to speak to your mental health team, contact your GP and ask for a referral - again, do not accept no for an answer; insist on the referral if your GP is hesitant.

Look to charities as well for support, such as the Alzheimer's Society, Dementia UK, and Young-Onset Dementia Network, just to name a few. Some of these charities have a help line that you can call for advice and guidance. There will probably be local charities that can help you with guidance as well as financial advice. These charities can support you in filling out the dreaded Personal

Independence Payment (PIP) or claiming benefits. For finances, work on the proviso that if you do not ask, you will not get.

If it is more specialised support you require, then have a word with your mental health team or your doctor. They can refer you to Social Services for a social worker or an occupational therapist. Again, do this as early as possible so that you can start to plan for the future rather than waiting for that crisis point.

Why a social worker? These will be able to point you in the right direction and assist you with some of the financial, housing, and benefits needs that you may have.

Why an occupational therapist? They will be able to assist you with your physical needs as the disease progresses.

In my experience, doing this as early as possible enables you to have the contacts that you will need later. It is true you may not need them fully now, but they can help you to prepare for what is to come.

Note: It is the NHS protocol that the Mental Health Services discharge you back to your doctor just one month after your diagnosis. When they ask, or they say they are going to do this, say: "No!! I want to remain under the Mental

Health Services." They may try and tell you that they must do this, but really, they do not have to do this. Ask them if they would discharge a person with cancer shortly after diagnosis.

Mental Health Services are the specialists in dementia care so why would they want to discharge you back to a doctor who is a general practitioner? It makes no sense at all and, frankly, is a shortfall when it comes to the NHS guidance for the Mental Health Services. Remember to say no; you have that right, but do so respectfully and in a calm voice. They are just doing their job and what they have been instructed to do.

State the reason for wanting to stay under the Mental Health Services; they are your gateway to more specialised support; for example, to psychologists, occupational services, nurses, medication, and social services, to name just a few things.

If you have been discharged by the Mental Health Services already and feel you need their support again, you do not need to go back to your doctor to get a referral. That can take ages. Contact the Mental Health Services direct. Because you have been diagnosed and they have cared for you before, you have that direct link back into the services - another value of getting diagnosed!

You cannot prepare for every eventuality because, for each person, dementia is different. We do not know how our brain will deteriorate, but being prepared can take a little of the stress and anxiety out of the situation for both you and for the loved one caring for you.

The key to good support now and later is having the lines of communications open with as many support networks as you can.

Do not forget to sort out your Will and your Health and Welfare LPA (Lasting Power of Attorney) as well as your financial LPA. Plan ahead! Some of these can be done for free through legal services linked to one of the charities mentioned above.

If you are the one caring, I suggest openly speaking to your loved one about what you would like to do and follow the same guidance above. You may face reluctance; I most certainly did when it came to my mom and dad. They thought they could manage this disease on their own and the needs of my mom would not be an issue. How wrong they were! As the disease progressed, more help was required, but because we did not build-up the contacts before, we found it ridiculously hard to get the help we needed. It felt like a constant battle to sometimes get even the simplest of advice and help. I will be honest; I did most of my research using the Internet and the Alzheimer's Society website. I am glad I did this because little was I to know that I would be using that same information for myself later...

Note: Young onset Dementia creates a whole host of unique challenges. Unfortunately, it becomes harder to get some support especially in the financial area. That is simply because you do not fall into the Government's misinformed definition of those with dementia, that is, those over the age of 65. As such, many of the support benefits will not apply to you, but if you do not ask, you will not get. You can only try. As unfair as it is, there is not much you can do if they say no. Welcome to my life!

Once you know whom to speak to or whom to go to for help and support, the help and support is there. Make use of it; you will need help and support whether you are the person living with or affected by dementia.

Note: You can get a lot of support from people going through the same or similar situations to yours, whether you are a person living with dementia or a carer.

Peer support should never be underrated; it can be invaluable. Being able to speak to people going through the same troubles you are facing, people who have been through or who are going through the acceptance stage will help you immensely. Such ones will have different tips regarding how they deal with things or the support they have in place. You may be able to help them as well with tips you have found work for you.

The support network you build up over time will help you avoid making rash, emotional decisions, but rather more calculated, focused decisions pertaining to what would be best for you, the person living with dementia, and your loved one who cares for you so dearly.

But no matter what others tell you. You need to be open and honest with yourself. Kicking the can down the road, so to speak, will only last so long before you reach crisis stage, and that is what we are trying to avoid by discussing these points early or as needed.

Our dear valued carers

I would like to say something to you, our valued carers, for a moment.

The above advice applies to you as well. You, too, can get support, and there are carer support groups you can contact. The Mental Health Services are there for you, as well as the social workers and nurses.

People living with dementia have to deal with their symptoms, and as the dementia progresses, that's all we have to deal with as everything else blurs into the peripheral. But as carers, you deal with all the symptoms and the challenges that bring, including the mood swings, but you also have to deal with all the finances and those peripheral things as well. Not to forget your own problems and concerns.

Knowing what that feels like, I say this:

CARE FOR YOURSELF!

You are no good to anyone if you are struggling as well. That is why that support network is so important. Use it as you need it, but do so before it comes to the point where you cannot cope. Your health and mental wellbeing is just as important, if not more important, than the loved one diagnosed.

So, care for yourself. Take time for yourself. Allow yourself to de-stress and unwind. That could be just taking an hour or so and going for coffee alone or with friends, or a night out, going shopping or to the pub. Whatever you enjoy that allows you to unwind, do it. If you do not, dementia becomes so all-encompassing it will cause you damage physically, emotionally, or both. Remember, take care of yourself, take time for yourself. It is not being selfish; it is vital for you to do this.

I never really appreciated that when caring for my mom and dad. You just do it because you love them and want to help and care for them, almost on autopilot. If you do not care for them, then who does? I never gave much thought to myself. But now that I am diagnosed, I appreciate both sides of the coin and have come to realise how much more difficult it is to care for someone living with dementia than it is to live with it. Do not get me wrong, living with this disease is hard, but to be a carer is harder and with so much more to deal with.

So, to my dad, who was my mom's primary carer and to my lovely wife and son, I would like to say a big thank you for what you did for my mom and what you are doing for me now. I know that mom would have been greatly appreciative and thankful for all that you did for her, dad, and the sacrifice you made right to the bitter end. I would like to show my appreciation and thankfulness to my beautiful wife and son as well. I know I may not always say so or, even due to the mood swings, may say things or do things that annoy you or that you find hard to cope with, but I will always be grateful for all that you do for me now and will do later.

If you have no family

Sadly, some do not have family to call on or to care for them when struggling, and to those whom I know who are in this situation, I tip my hat too. I do not think I could cope with this disease on my own and all of life's challenges as well.

If you are in this situation, follow the advice above. Many I speak to find that finances are the hardest struggle.

A word of warning here: we have all heard of those who take advantage of vulnerable people, and money makes people do weird and out-of-character things. Choose a friend that you trust to handle or help you with your finances or that can help you make health decisions. Get legal support for this to cover your own back, so to speak. LPAs are invaluable in this case.

If, however, you do not have that trusted friend, then speak to your bank and explain the situation. There will be someone at the bank who is trained in speaking and dealing with people living with dementia, and you can request that person to speak to. They can assign someone who is liable under the law to help you manage your finances, so you have the safety of knowing that. You can also speak to your social worker, and they can assign someone as well. I do not think

I would go the social worker route, but that is my preference. You can also speak to the individual companies you have dealings with and explain your situation to them and see what they offer.

Either way and whatever support you need, do not do it alone or be afraid to ask for help. Be it that of finances, help around the house, cooking. There is help out there for you – get it, get the help you need, do not struggle in silence. This disease is hard enough to live with!

Though you have no immediate family or family that are willing to care for you, there are friends out there that will take up this role with a smile; there are support networks.

YOU ARE NEVER ALONE! We are all here for you.

Key Points:

Dementia affects everyone who faces it.

You will have challenging emotions and have many questions, this is natural.

Remember to stay in the present.

Speak openly about your feelings and emotions; peer support is invaluable here.

Plan for the future.

YOUR NOTES AND THOUGHTS:

Weighing up the positives and negatives for now and the future

Based on what we have just discussed, and you feel emotionally secure, perhaps now is a good time to think about the positives and negatives of the future.

I called this section "weighing up the positives and negatives for now and the future" but what realistically are the positives of dementia? I can think of many negatives...

But there can be positives for my future. As far as I can, and as independently as I can, I would like the future to be in my hands.

Do not be afraid to adapt. By understanding your needs, your concerns, your issues, and your problems it is easier to adapt. I know, for example, that I have balance issues, so when my balance is off, then I will use a walking aid. At first, it took a bit of getting used to. I felt a bit embarrassed, but it helped, so I took the reasoning, "Who cares what others think?" I also found that due to my age, people did not know or could identify that I have dementia, and this resulted in some saying nasty words or getting impatient with me. I found a small badge that said I had dementia. I wear that badge now wherever I go, and it helps people who are not ignorant realise the struggles that I will be having or the reason for me being a bit slower, and so show me the patience that I need.

I have also found that due to spatial awareness issues, I have smashed a few glasses and broken a few plates. To adapt, I have changed from using glasses to now using plastic glasses that look just as smart. I have also changed the colour of my plates from white to grey. This not only enables me to see the plate but also to see the food on the plate. The normal silver cutlery was a problem for me as well, so I switched those to coloured ones. Minor changes, but it makes a world of difference.

There are other areas that I have adapted but it is all about knowing yourself, acknowledging where you need support, and which support you need. I have already mentioned the use of Alexa and digital calendars and how they help me keep my day organised.

What I am really saying here is that we can turn a negative into a positive by just being able to adapt. We no longer have to choose to look at things the way some feel we should, that once we can't do something then that's it. I am saying, based on my experience, that by being prepared to adapt, we can still do things. Perhaps we cannot do them the way we used to, or maybe not even as efficiently as we did before, but we can still do things, albeit a little differently.

To keep the future in your hands requires that we think and plan ahead. Let people know what your wishes are. Your Will, the LPA's, and advanced directives all make your wishes explicit. These documents are there not only as a protection but also to inform your loved ones how and even when you would like things to be done when you can no longer make that decision. It is taking one step into the future circle while keeping the other foot firmly planted in the present circle.

When we think about it, positives and negatives are really what we make of them and the current situation we find ourselves in. For example, being diagnosed with dementia has meant that I need more support in certain things, but if you have people who love you and are willing to support you, I see that as a positive. I have always tried to look on the bright side of things despite it being very difficult sometimes to find that bright side, and that's what dementia will do to you. It will make you think that there are no bright sides. There are bright sides, but they must come from within you and from those who support you.

Due to my diagnosis and my desire to help others in a similar situation, I took it upon myself to be more engaged in volunteering for various charities specifically the Alzheimer's Society, Young Dementia Network, Bradford University. Doing so has given me another positive, that of friends, people who understand what I am going through. Some of these are diagnosed, and others are staff who have taken me under their wing and supported me on my journey. There is one specific friend whose name I will not mention, but she will know who she is. It showed me that sometimes you can find support and friendship in unlikely places, support and friendship that will help you on your journey.

I had to adapt here, too, especially when in meetings. I found that wearing a lanyard that identifies me as having dementia helped. The lanyard had my name on it and stated that I have dementia and requested that people be patient. This helped in two ways. Firstly, it enabled people to know my name, and so when they spoke to me, they addressed me by name, making it easier for me to identify that they were speaking to me. Secondly, it enabled people to know that I have dementia and that my thought processes or my speech may be a little bit slower than normal. I found those that I worked with to be more patient as a result.

Another positive would be that of staying in your own home. You are familiar with your surroundings. Most times, you know where things are. Silly things, that we would normally take for granted, for example, where are the light switches? These are things that in our own home, we know and are familiar with. It is also where our memories are, especially if we have been in the home for a long time.

Some of the advice that you may get will tell you to stay in your own home for as long as you possibly can because this is the best thing for you. They base this theory mostly on what we have just discussed: familiarity with your own home, as well as the memories that you have built up there. In my opinion, this thinking is flawed; allow me to explain my reasoning in the next chapter.

So, dealing with a negative or something that you are currently struggling with is really down to how you view or feel about that struggle and your willingness to adapt. Change is something you will have to do as the disease progresses, whether you like it or not, so making that change as early as possible will make it easier to come to terms with or get used to doing things in a different way while you still can manage that change and comprehend why you needed to adapt. It also minimises the frustration for you and for those caring for you.

You will know by now that frustration causes tensions and feelings of uselessness. Do not struggle unnecessarily when it is within your power to change and adapt.

There will come times when you cannot adapt or make a change due to the progression of the disease. When that happens, ask yourself, "Is what I am trying to do important? Will it make a big difference if I do not do it?"

If the answer is no, then walk away, so to speak. Leave it for another day or ask for assistance. I have found it is better to do that rather than get frustrated and snap at those who love me. Sometimes though, due to how I feel, that still does happen from time to time. I can only try my hardest to control those feelings as best as I can.

I think I might have mentioned before that this disease is not easy to live with.

All you can do is try your best to make changes and adapt. Remember though, try speaking to the peer support network you have built up and see what they do to cope with what you are struggling with. You may pick up some tips that could work for you or your loved one.

Where there is a will, there is a way. Until there isn't.

Key Points:

There are many negatives to having dementia, but with a little help and a lot of determination, it is possible to turn a negative into a positive.

Try your best to stay positive and remain in the present.

Learning to accept and adapt will serve you well.

Accept support.

YOUR NOTES AND THOUGHTS:

Living Situation

Staying in your current home

In some situations, in fact most situations, you may be able to stay in your own home with a few modifications or perhaps additional support.

It is true we get attached to our homes, especially if we have been there for many years or seen our children grow up there; staying there for as long as you possibly can makes sense. But remember, we are trying to avoid a crisis situation; we are trying to look at things and make decisions before they become a problem. So, consider this: what if, for some reason, the home starts to cause you stress and anxiety? Perhaps you keep having falls. Then it would be time to discuss whether staying in your own home is a good thing.

I am not saying at this point that you need to consider moving, but perhaps you need to consider modifications to your home or arrange additional support to help you manage. Whatever the case, whatever you discuss with your loved ones, know that this will be an emotional subject. Be honest with yourself and with others, and be patient.

If you know the type and the subtype of your dementia, then plan around that. Perhaps you should consider spatial awareness or visual impairment. [Visual impairment doesn't imply that there are problems with your eyes. In the case of dementia, it can often mean that your eyes can see well, but your brain cannot compute what it is seeing. For example, a carpet that is a dark colour could look like a hole, a shiny surface may look wet, and colours that are of similar shade will seem to blend together]. You may also have to consider the memory issue; where things are, where things are put. This may seem logical to you as a carer, but for a person with dementia, it can cause great anxiety and stress if things are moved or not put in the same place.

Things around your home that were once easy to find, easy to access, and easy to remember may, over time, become a problem. So, as time progresses and the disease progresses, be prepared to adapt as you go. I took the view that I would do as much preparation as possible to try and get used to the things that I was adapting.

Some of the things that I adapted were, for example, the lights. I would constantly forget to switch the lights off or, in some cases, not know where the light switches were, even though I had been in the house for nearly 20 years. As I had Alexa in the house, I thought it would be easier to change to smart light bulbs. This meant that in most of the rooms, the lights were voice-activated, so if I forgot, I could just speak.

Another problem area for me was the depth perception of the stairs. I found myself tripping up the stairs because I could not judge the depth of the rise of the stairs. To adapt, I changed the carpet, carpeting the stairs but not the rise. The rise I painted in a distinct colour. I then fell or tripped much less. While we are talking about stairs and my balance issues, I also found it helpful to put handrails on both sides of the stairs.

I made other adaptations to help with the spatial awareness. I found door architraves - the frames around a door - to be a problem if they had different shapes. Simply put, I would walk into them and hurt my shoulder or face. To prevent this, I went with a simple round edge architrave and then painted them, as well as the door, in a bright colour. My walls were beige in colour, so I painted the door and its frames bright white.

A little tip here if you do struggle with spatial awareness or colours: take a picture of the thing that is causing you a problem, then turn that picture into black and white. If the item causing you a problem and its surrounding areas appear either all white or all black, that is what your brain sees and there is the problem! Change one of them to a distinct colour so that one object becomes black and the other object becomes white; that will provide a good contrast that your brain can identify. A very smart occupational therapist helped me with this.

Put different aids in place in the kitchen. As the carer, remember to put things in the same place, remember the contrast, and have something that will cover the hob for when it might be hot.

These are all minor changes, but they make an enormous difference, which will allow you to stay in your home longer. Remember, adapt as you go!

Some of these changes may seem so small and insignificant if you are the carer, but if it makes life simpler for the loved one with dementia, then really, what is the harm other than you having to get used to doing things slightly differently? If a person living with dementia is happy and content, then generally, the mood changes are minimal, and it becomes easier for you both to accept what is happening. It also gives you more time to focus on what really matters: time together!

The financial strain on making these adaptations should be something to also consider seriously. Does the cost justify the adaptation? Will the adaptation improve the value of the house? Will I be putting more money into the house than it is worth?

We considered changing the garage to a downstairs bedroom; upon investigation, this would cost a lot of money and not add any value to the house. So, doing small adaptations that enabled me to move to and from the bedroom upstairs was more cost-effective. The house only had one bathroom, which was upstairs; this, too, was a problem. So, we decided that we would spend some of the money on putting in a downstairs wet room. This meant I did not have to go up and down the stairs as often throughout the day. It also meant that I could shower without having to step in and out of a bath, and it added value to the house. Three problems, one solution.

I would like to mention support at this point. You will find that there is very little support out there regarding making adaptations to your house. The occupational therapists will be able to help with certain adaptations that will help you move around better, but when it comes to building work or modifications to your home, there is very little to no support. There are some charities that might be able to help you with a grant, but these are few and far between, and you have to qualify for them. One of the downsides of young onset dementia is that a lot of times, the criteria is based on your age and, so we do not qualify. You can however, if you decide to do home modifications or building work, claim the VAT back on certain things. Most times the contractor that you use will be able to help you with this; there is simply a form that you sign that they then send off to HMRC. This allows you to get the building work done without having to pay VAT. Because dementia is classed as a disability, you will qualify for this. However, not all modifications or building work qualifies - you can check on the HMRC website to see which ones do.

With that in mind and keeping your future in your own hands, perhaps a decision to move earlier might be better. That is the way I looked at it, but I only made that decision after I had exhausted all other options for staying in my own home and once my wife and I agreed that this was the best action.

When to consider moving

In the case that staying in your own home is not possible, and you or your loved one feel that it might be best to change accommodation, then be open and honest about how you feel and the reasons why you feel a change is needed. Again, this can be an area where emotions can run high. Quite often, you are asking to move the person out of their family home, and that generally never goes down well initially.

Be patient, show kindness, and listen to both sides of the story. If you can make the decision together, this will always end up in a happier family arrangement. Sadly, in some cases, this is not possible. As the disease progresses and the person deteriorates, the ability to make these decisions fades, and it can be down to you to make the very difficult decision, a decision that will always tug at your heartstrings.

In the case with my mom, my dad was very reluctant, for obvious reasons, to put my mom into care even though he was struggling, and his health was starting to deteriorate because of the strain that caring for somebody with dementia can put on you. After an open conversation with my dad, we decided that it was in his and my mum's best interest to place her in care. It was perhaps the hardest decision I've ever had to make.

In my case, once we had agreed that our house was no longer suitable and that it would cost too much to make it so, another possibility was needed. It was a matter of trying to decide what would be best. We could buy a bungalow; we could buy another house that would work for us. In some cases, as with my mum, it was deciding which care home to move her into.

Choosing a Suitable Home

My wife and I eventually came to the realisation that staying in our current home was not going to be the best choice. It was going to be too costly to modify, which would not be the best use of our money.

Separation was never an option, so whatever we decided to do, we were always going to be together. While we can be together and my wife can manage looking after me, we will stay together.

We looked at some bungalows. Most we looked at required a lot of work to bring them to the standard we were looking for. I will be honest again here and say that bungalows are expensive and few and far between, but it seemed the logical option. We did not see the point of buying another house with stairs as they were the initial problem for me. We considered looking for a house with a downstairs bedroom but then thought that the rest of the house would not be used if there were stairs; that didn't seem logical to me.

I will add at this point that you will find very little support here, either financially or otherwise, not even support to move. Some councils used to offer this service, but as the budget squeeze took its toll, a lot of these services were withdrawn.

Social housing is a possibility. It is a long-winded process that takes a lot of time and frustration, but if this is your only way and you qualify for it, it is certainly worth looking at. I have found, as have others that I have spoken to with young onset dementia, that most of the time, you will not qualify as things stand, especially if your partner is still working. But if you do, certainly give this a go. The occupational therapist and social services can help with this, so have a word with them first.

As I had built up a good network of people I could call upon, I let some know of my concerns and my thoughts about moving. A local dementia charity that I had worked with that also supports the Young Onset Dementia group in our area gave me a suggestion, an idea that we had never considered: moving into Alms housing.

Alms housings are a charity-owned housing that are for people who are struggling with various issues. Some of these are supported or assisted-living accommodations. The housing we looked at was supported living, meaning that there is a support worker on hand during the day and a call facility for the night should you need them because of, for example, a fall. The qualifications to get into one of these houses are listed on the individual charity's website or on the Alms Housing website.

The dementia charity that helped me (Hospital of God) was prepared to even make alterations to the cottage at their cost. The layout of the cottage was not suitable for someone with balance issues or for a person living with dementia. Needless doors and walls; lighting causing shadows; large heaters that stuck out into the room, all of which were causing me confusion, instability, and trip hazards when moving through the cottage.

After consultation with ourselves and the building contractors, they removed the walls and doors and changed the lighting and heating. They were prepared to do or find a solution to whatever was needed.

They even allowed us to replace the kitchen, bedroom wardrobes, and wet room with more modern fittings and fixtures. These, along with the decorating, we did at our cost as this is something my wife and I wanted rather than needed.

We will be forever grateful for their understanding and readiness to take the opportunity to help someone living with young-onset dementia when so many would not have. We really cannot thank you all enough for the great vision you have to help myself and other people living with dementia.

An added bonus for me is that there is also a highly rated care home on the property, which will be handy for my next move.

It meant downsizing, which we were prepared to do. It was not much cheaper either in comparison to the mortgage, but it was still the best move we have made. I am much happier and more stable here in the new cottage. I also have help should I need it later. Knowing that my wife will have a home after I have moved into care or passed away and knowing that I have the care and support that I will need puts my mind at ease. Now, I can concentrate on living the best way I can.

So, consider all the facts before you make any decisions. Get all the advice, help, and support you can - this will help you make a decision that will benefit you and your family.

Consider not only what you will need now but also in the future. The future is uncertain. You cannot know for certain what it will be like. My theory is that you can never be too prepared. Do research on your type of dementia, as we have mentioned before and speak to others who have been through this. This will help you paint a good picture of your future and what you or your loved ones will need.

There is no need to make the same mistakes others have by thinking it will be different for you when so many living with dementia or who have lived through it say otherwise. Is that not the very definition of stupidity? Doing the same thing but expecting a different result!

Based on what information you find and what others say who have lived through it, plan.

Planning for your future early can only reduce the frustration later for everyone. It will not stop the frustration, but the aim of this advice is to help you reduce that stress while you can still do so.

If that means moving or modifying your home, do so early enough to get what you want out of it. Letting it get to a crisis point will only lead to resentment and arguments.

Memories are not in brick and mortar. They are in your heart, deep within you. Sentiment can cloud judgment. It is very hard to do but try putting emotions aside when making these types of decisions. Not easy I know, I have been there, but it is necessary.

Planning means you can do it all together; everyone knows what you want and when you want these things to happen.

In my opinion, do this as early as possible, but only if you have passed the acceptance stage and feel your mind is clear enough to do so.

Care Home

Let us consider the discussion of moving your loved one into a care home or choosing to move into a care home.

My mom had reached late-stage dementia by this point and was having issues with eating and drinking. She was not sleeping well and was keeping my dad awake, too. I was getting calls at silly hours of the night informing me that my mom was becoming aggressive with my dad because she did not know where she was or even who he was. For some reason, my mom always knew who I was, and so I could calm her down and my dad too. She was also double-incontinent. All of these things placed a great strain on my dad; he was really suffering. Even so, he wanted to continue to care for my mom. But it was too much for him. I had to help him realise that it was time for specialised care in a care home.

As I said before, this will be one of the hardest decisions you will ever have to make.

Be aware though, that sometimes this decision is taken out of your hands in that the social workers or the NHS will decide for you. That is not the best outcome, so it is better to try and make this decision for yourself before it gets to that point.

The social worker and the occupational therapist will be able to give you guidance on this, but this will only work if you are open and honest with them.

In the case of my mom, we left it too late, if I'm being honest. I allowed my dad's feelings to cloud my judgement. We promised my mom that we would only move her into care as a final resort. I feel we stuck to that promise, but it came at a price, and now the social worker was insisting that it was time to move her into a care home. The social worker was kind enough to let us choose which one; he very kindly gave us time to do this but with an ultimatum that if we did not, then they would.

Choosing a care home was exceedingly difficult to do. I did not have all the information that we have now. It came as quite a surprise that not all care homes can adequately care for people with dementia. It also came as a surprise that not all care homes had the same quality of care. This meant that we had to visit care homes and ask questions until, eventually, we chose one that we thought would be best for my mom.

Thankfully, this turned out to be the case. The care home that she went into had great staff, and they would do anything for my mom or for us when we visited. They would allow my dad to go daily, and he could stay all day. They would give him food and drinks as needed. The dementia area of the care home was a controlled zone, which meant that my mom would be safe and could not wander out. It also had a nice courtyard, which allowed her to go outside safely.

A note you might want to consider here. Each care home has its own doctor that they will call in if they feel the resident needs medical attention. This doctor will most likely not be the one that has cared for your loved one through their journey so far. This created a problem for us as the doctor that was called out for my mom knew nothing about dementia, and you could see that by the way she was talking to my mom and the questions she was asking that she was never going to get a response to in a month of Sundays! Which I must say, I found very strange considering that this was the dementia area of the care home. You would think a doctor who knew about dementia would be called, but this was not the case. So, you may want to ask if you can still use the family doctor and check if the doctor is prepared to go out to see your loved one. They have all the history and know your loved one well.

If this is not possible, perhaps you could make an appointment with their doctor and ascertain for yourself what they are like with patients and how much they know about dementia care.

I was not impressed with this doctor and, so I asked her to leave and called in the mental health team to offer help to my mom and the care home. The mental health team was more than willing to assist me even though it was a bit further to travel.

Sadly, my mom deteriorated rapidly and was very quickly placed in palliative care. Here again, the care home staff was very considerate and caring. Upon my mum's death, they took care of everything and allowed us to stay with her as long as we needed to.

Take time, do not rush the decision as to which care home you are going to choose and if you can avoid doing this in a crisis stage like we found ourselves in, all the better. If possible, allow the person with dementia to be involved in the decision, though I acknowledge this is not always possible. If you can do it with the person and they are not too far advanced, then it gives the person time to settle in and to get used to their surroundings.

What you want to try and avoid is moving them into a care home only to find it is not up to your standard of care and then have to move them again. This will cause the person to deteriorate much more quickly.

Also, keep in mind the financial implications of a care home. Social services will decide what percentage they will cover and how much you will have to pay - this could be in the thousands! This often comes down to the type of care you will need. The more independent the person is, the more you will have to pay. With my mom they said a 50/50 split. My dad did not have that kind of money, and my mom was now in the late stages of dementia, requiring a lot of care. We pushed back, and eventually, with a bit of fighting and a good social care worker we got the 100% cover.

The moral here is to fight. Do not accept the first contract they produce (unless you can afford it, but that is up to you).

Tip! Today, we have a wealth of information on care homes. Make use of that information when deciding on which care home to choose. The Care Quality Commission [CQC], in conjunction with Healthwatch England, give care homes a rating. The CQC look at the quality of care, from medical staffing levels, training of staff, the condition of the building, and the adequacy of the rooms to other valuable information that they are mandated to audit on. Healthwatch England investigates what family, friends, and residents say about the care home, the staff, the food, and any other information you may find valuable.

Using this information gives you a more rounded view of each care home. All this information can be found by looking at their websites. You can, of course, armed with all this information, do your own additional investigation when visiting the care home. Speak to the staff, speak to the residents, ask to taste the food. Generally, most care homes will allow you to do this.

I will not lie, though, after moving my mom into a care home, I felt really rubbish. I felt bad for my dad, and I felt like I had abandoned my mum, even though I knew it was the best and the right thing to do. Nonetheless, the guilt weighed heavily. I just had to keep reminding myself that this was the right thing to do for my mum and for the care and stability of my dad.

Key Points:

Consider all your options carefully and where you can include the person living with dementia. But remember, this will be emotional for you all.

Take sentiment out of the situation the best you can when considering a care home move.

Do your homework. Don't be afraid to ask and research the care home you are considering.

If you decide to stay at your own home, be prepared to adapt.

Be open and honest about your struggles and what might be best for you and your loved ones.

Memories are in you, not in the brick and mortar.

Moving to somewhere more suitable may help with being independent for a bit longer.

Accept support and advice when considering what to do next.

YOUR NOTES AND THOUGHTS:

Staying active physically and mentally

Staying physically and mentally active is important, irrespective of whether you have dementia or not. The benefits far outweigh any negatives.

Other benefits for those living with dementia that have been noted on the Alzheimer's Society UK website (2024) are:

"Improving physical fitness - maintaining strong muscles and flexible joints can help people maintain independence for longer.

Improving the ability to dress, clean, cook and perform other daily activities (as these may be performed more effectively if someone is fitter or more supple).

Helping to keep bones strong and reducing the risk of osteoporosis (a disease that affects the bones, making them weak and more likely to break).

Improving cognition - recent studies have shown that exercise may improve memory and slow down mental decline.

Improving sleep.

Providing opportunities for social interaction and reducing the feeling of isolation.

Reducing the risk of falls by improving strength and balance.

Improving confidence.

Increasing self-esteem.

Improving mood."

Alzheimer's Society 2024 - https://www.alzheimers.org.uk/get-support/daily-living/exercise

Keeping physically active can be easier said than done, though, when living with dementia, and if you are caring for someone, then it comes down to time. But it is not impossible.

Keep in mind the type of dementia you have, as well as how far advanced you are, when choosing what types of exercise to undertake. The last thing you want is to hurt yourself trying to do something your mind or body cannot handle; that defeats the objective. Know your limitations and adapt as you can.

All my life, I was physically active. If there was a sport, I would be playing it. I would regularly do weight training. But as time went on, I found that engaging in some of these sports, or doing free weight training, was becoming challenging both physically and mentally.

I wrongly thought that forcing my body and mind to do what it has always done was the correct way; after all, this is what a lot of science and dementia specialists were saying. They were wrong! I did a lot of damage to my body, including tearing muscles and bone fractures, as I lost count of my repetitions or forgot to warm up correctly, and I lost my balance a few times.

I did not give up, though; I found ways to adapt. I use a treadmill that has barriers so I can keep my balance. Rather than doing free weights, I use machines, and where I can sit, I will.

I have also found that less active sports are better now. I found playing bowls, ten-pin bowling, and table tennis better for me. It uses a lot of muscle groups as well as brain power. Darts is also good for hand-to-eye coordination and brain power, though not physically challenging. Swimming is good if you can. Walking for just 10 minutes a day helps greatly.

Things such as gardening, housework, and moving your legs and arms while sitting all count towards keeping active.

After finding I had time on my hands, I discovered that I enjoy gardening. I redesigned my garden to have raised beds to make it safer for me. I have always enjoyed working with my hands, especially with wood so not only did I design but carried out the hard landscaping as well.

Note: If you are going to use power tools, be smart. If you are not feeling cognitively good or your balance is off, then do not use these tools! It will be dangerous; leave it for another day. Never use the tools on your own - always let someone know what you are doing for safety reasons.

When we sold our house and moved, I lost the garden. Thankfully, the charity that I moved to realise the importance of getting outside as well as how therapeutic gardening can be. Outside my back door is a grassed courtyard used by all the residents and other support groups. They said I could do what I wanted in the garden.

I have designed a dementia-friendly garden, which the residents and the charity approve of, and I have started the hard landscaping and planting. I enjoy it.

I do have to make adaptions as I go. I can no longer remember the measurements before I cut, so I write them down on the wood. Measure twice, cut once, they say! I measure 15 times and cut once and still sometimes get it wrong, ha ha. I do not let that stop me, though.

I would often put my tools somewhere and then could not find them again, needlessly wandering around to find something. I now put things in one place. It may mean moving back and forth a bit, but once I have finished with a tool or the tape measure, I will put it back in the same place. Keeping everything together helps me be a little bit more organised.

I also clear up after myself as I go. This helps with my balance and visual perception.

Reducing my frustration levels, using less brain power and trying to find things helps me do the tasks I enjoy. Plus, a little help from my beautiful wife when I need it, even if it is them checking on me or making sure I drink.

The key is to be reasonable, use common sense, and if you struggle or feel unwell, stop and rest. But do what you enjoy, and do not be afraid to start new things. You might be surprised what you enjoy or can do. Dementia does not spell an end to learning or trying new things.

Mental activity is just as good as physical activity.

Using your brain can only be a good thing despite the challenges it poses. Does it slow the progression of the dementia? Science is still out on that one. My thought is that it cannot hurt to try. I am not the sort to just lay down and let things happen. I will try, then adapt, and then try again until I can no longer do so.

My mom loved to do jigsaw puzzles. For as long as I can remember, there was always a puzzle on the go. Heaven help you if you try put a piece in, ha ha.

As the dementia progressed, she started to struggle more and more. The puzzle size got smaller, then the pieces got bigger until it became more frustrating than enjoyable for her.

My mom was never that good with technology, but we found some jigsaw puzzle apps that she could manage, which we loaded onto a tablet for her. She adapted but never gave up.

Eventually, the dementia advanced so much that even the adaptations no longer worked. What do you do then?

Some doctors and dementia specialists will tell you to force them to carry on, in this case, with the puzzles. That caused so many arguments and tears.

They are wrong!

Remember what is happening to the brain - it is shrinking! Capacity to do things is dying. We would never ask a person who has lost a limb to get up and walk unaided, would we? The capacity to do so is no longer available, so that would be very cruel.

The same is true with the brain. If the capacity is no longer there, you cannot force the person to do something they just cannot do anymore. It is cruel and frustrating for everyone.

But, like the person who has lost a limb, it does not mean the person can no longer do other things or get around. There are aids out there to help them. Even with dementia, the brain is a very smart and powerful organ. We can find other things to do that the brain will accept.

My mom found that she could colour, and she enjoyed it. So, we helped her with that, either on paper or on an app. It is something I found I enjoy as well. I colour using apps and find it relaxing.

Others have found they can paint, draw, make jewellery or cards, or do word or number puzzles. Whatever it is that you choose, you keep your brain active, which can only be of benefit.

Remember, adapt as needed, and when it is no longer fun and becomes frustrating, try something else. Keep trying.

The time will come for all of us with dementia when we do become that person people think about when we mention dementia. That is a very late stage, and we are not there yet. Until then, keep physically and mentally active as much as you can, within reason.

If you need support, speak to your loved ones or the occupational therapist, and they will be able to guide and assist you in keeping active.

Key points:

There are many benefits to staying mentally and physically active, but do so within your limits and rest as needed.

Find a hobby, but be prepared to adapt when required.

You can still learn new things.

Have fun whatever you choose to do.

Accept the support you need.

YOUR NOTES AND THOUGHTS:

Volunteering. Why, how, when, and for whom?

When I was told I could no longer work, and to be honest, I was not in the right headspace anyway, it was a real blow.

I was 47 at the time, still prime working age. Once I had accepted what was happening and dealt with my mom's passing, I found myself wanting to do something to help my wife deal with the situation we found ourselves in, and I still do.

But realistically, I know that if a person being diagnosed is being put on ill health or retired, then what chance will I have of getting a job after having been diagnosed? I am right; as soon as people know you have dementia, you don't get a look in, even if you are qualified for the position.

I am doing things and keeping busy, as you have read, but I am still not contributing to the household, and that is getting me down. This is not a case of chivalry. Seeing my wife take everything on her shoulders is difficult to accept when we have always worked together in running the house and regarding financial matters.

Even though I have resigned myself to this is how it will be. This still does not make it any easier.

Someone suggested volunteering. My first thought was shaking a container and asking for money for charity. I thought that was not for me, but then the person said this was not what they were referring to. They explained about all the options available and that you could volunteer as much or as little time as you like.

This person was diagnosed, and so I had a look into it, thinking if she can do it, then so could I. This is what I found.

Most dementia charities are looking for volunteers, so you are not restricted in choice. I wanted a charity that had values I could relate too and a charity that would see me, not my dementia nor my story. A charity that would allow me to use my skills as a project manager and business analyst.

What I found is that most of these charities want me to tell my story, which they could use to get donations that, in turn, helps to fund the charity that offers the support or research grants.

Like I said earlier, I wanted to be more than my story but thought that this was a way in. I would suggest this will be a good place to start if volunteering is what you are looking to do. You can complete a volunteer form found on their website, and they will contact you to set up a chat in order to find out more about you.

Note: telling your story can be emotionally and physically challenging and tiring. It can take a lot out of you, more than I anticipated. You will talk about your highs and lows and how you and your family are managing. Emotional stuff! I would not suggest doing this if you have not accepted your diagnosis and your future. I have seen people breakdown and find it very hard to continue as a result. A few times I was brought to tears talking about things and explaining how I was feeling. Be prepared for this. At the same time, if you choose a charity that sees you as a person, which most do, then they are trained for such emotional discussions. They will be kind, empathetic, and supportive. They will allow you to go at your own pace, even if this takes a few sessions.

I thought there must be more than this when volunteering? I raised the question with the person who was interviewing me. She told me there are a lot of things you can get involved in.

Alzheimer's Society, Alzheimer's Research UK (yes, they are separate charities), and NIHR, just to name a handful, are looking for volunteers with lived experience (diagnosed, carer, or former carer) to help advise with their research grant application process. I will say this is very interesting and very rewarding.

At first, I was apprehensive because science is not my forte. But actually, there was nothing to worry about. All of the research applications are sent in lay review format (that is common English to you and me). Not all the applications are science-based either - you can choose to see applications for care, for example, rather than science.

You also get a chance to interact with the researchers as well. Ask them questions, let them ask you questions and look for suggestions. The early career researchers, to me, are the best to get involved with. They are so eager to learn and interact. Training and speaking to them is always a pleasure.

The reason I find this so rewarding is because you can play your part in shaping the future of dementia research and, in turn, the future of dementia. Try it; you will see what I am talking about and why I am excited about this area of volunteering. Again, you can get involved as little or as much as you want. At any point in volunteering, you can always stop.

If this is not your cup of tea, you can look to get involved in fund raising and charity events.

You could look to be a trustee for a charity. I am a trustee and find this rewarding as well. I wanted to do this for a local charity, which I did for Dementia Friendly Hartlepool. After working with the Alzheimer's Society, I raised the question about whether they have a person diagnosed on the trustee board. They had discussed it previously, but the time was not right, they said. I asked what was wrong with the present. I am happy to say the first person diagnosed with dementia has now been appointed to the trustee board.

You could join steering groups and help shape the support people need, as well as policies and procedures, even at a national level. For this, I have found the Alzheimer's Society, Dementia UK, and Young Dementia Network to be the best. This line of work has led me to joining steering groups and committees such as policy, research, and communications committee for the Alzheimer's Society; Young Dementia Network steering group; Department of Health and Social Care dementia subgroup; Brain for Dementia Committee-Alzheimer's Research UK - just to name a few that I do work with. There are others as well.

You can do training at universities, colleges, care homes, NHS, and private businesses. I love training and public speaking. I know this is not for everyone, but if you can, give it a go. This, to me, is the more hands-on side of volunteering. I enjoy the face-to-face interaction. Being a part of a team that designed a new MSC for applied studies in dementia was a highlight, and now I'm enjoying being part of student training and evaluation for the Bradford University Centre for Applied Dementia Studies.

You can also do work with the NHS. They have "lived experience" volunteers helping them shape the future of the NHS. Some local services have Patient and Carer Participation Groups you can join. I joined the TEWV PCPG – a good bunch of people that have become great friends.

You can get involved in shaping the charity themselves by helping employees understand things about dementia. You could help with policies, procedures, aims and objectives if that is what you are good at. Not all charities do this, though, so you will need to ask, or if you are like me, you point out areas for improvement and help them make the necessary changes. You will have to do this gently, as no one likes to be told that they should or need to improve. You may meet resistance, I certainly did, but if you show your value and your willingness to get your hands dirty, they appreciate the help and guidance...I think. Seriously though, they do!

You could choose to get involved in medical or therapeutic trials. There are many available testing new equipment, new medication, etc. Do some research on this and do your homework on what you're testing, as well as what happens during and after the trial. Do not be afraid to walk away if this trial is not for you. If it is something you are already doing, then you are doing a good job and should be praised for it. There are not enough people that do this type of volunteering. Perhaps it's something you could consider.

This is what you will find when volunteering: no matter what type of volunteering you choose, you will make friends, and some of them will become good friends. Some can become part of your support network, as it is an excellent way to meet people who can help you when you need it.

Volunteering has taken me all over England and even from time to time overseas.

Volunteering has also given me a job. I view it as work and take it just as seriously. It differs, though, from paid work in that I can say no to something that I don't want to get involved in, or if I am going through a rough patch, I can walk away from it for a while until I feel strong enough again.

Volunteering did not solve the issue I have with getting paid to help support my wife, but it is a start. I am currently helping a charity look at ways in which they can employ people diagnosed and what that would look like, but there is a lot to consider if we want to get it right and sustainable. Watch this space!

Note: some charities and researchers will want to pay you for your time and effort. That is very kind of them, but there are things you need to consider before accepting such payments, especially if you are on benefits.

Accepting payment does not affect your Personal Independent Payments (PIP), so if that is all you get, then you can accept what you want. Even if you do go back to work at some point, PIP is not affected. Watch your savings, though.

If, on the other hand, you receive any type of means-tested benefit, then accepting a payment can affect those benefits. Unfortunately, the government does not appreciate what we have to go through as a volunteer, they just look at the money.

You are allowed to be paid up to about £140 a week for volunteer work as long as it is for no longer than 16 hours a week (this was the case at the time of writing). Anything over this and your benefits for that week can be stopped, or you could be asked to pay it back. It does not work on averages either; it is week by week.

This means that you can accept some payments but perhaps not all. That will be up to you. Sometimes, I will accept payment. Other times, I do not (even if I am nowhere near the allowed limit). If it is from a Pharma company, I will take payment; they are made of money, haha, but some charities are struggling and, so I will not accept payment from them. That is my personal choice.

If you choose to volunteer, you need to let the Department of Health and Welfare know. You do this by giving them a call or going to visit an office. There is a form you will need to complete. This protects you in case someone reports you or you are suspected of working. It covers your back and is law.

If you choose to accept payment, then you also need to let HMRC know. Again, this protects you, and that is the law. Any tax that is paid as a result of working will be paid back to you by HMRC at the end of the tax year as long as you do not exceed your personal tax threshold. You do not need to do anything, the HMRC will do this automatically if you have informed them.

Trying to hide it from the DWP or HMRC is not worth the risk. They are allowed to, and randomly do, monitor your accounts. Let them know it is quick and easy to do. The man I spoke to was polite and praised me for doing the work, and a note was added to my file. Every now and then, I get a form asking me who I worked with for this financial year, and that's it.

Just be aware of how much payment you accept each week and keep an eye on any savings you might have. An additional note here: Be aware that savings allowance between PIP and other benefits vary.

Volunteering is a way to give back. You may feel, after going through the diagnosis process and perhaps based on how you have been dealt with, that they do not deserve anything back. If so, then I put this to you, how can you expect it to improve if we do not volunteer and guide them?

Volunteering keeps you busy, keeps your mind active, and helps you feel as though you are contributing to something bigger than you.

I accept that a lot of what I am doing I will never see the benefits of, but my view is that if it helps the next person have a better diagnosis process, better support and after care, better social care, better medication and remove the postcode lottery from dementia, then we are doing our bit for a better future for those living with, and caring for people with, dementia.

I know I will not be able to volunteer for much longer, but at least I can say I did my bit. I did what I could.

Remember, you can choose what you want to get involved with, you can choose who you want to get involved with, and you can choose how much time you want to volunteer for. You can walk away at any time or take a break if needed. Let your charity contact know that you are doing this.

Volunteering is in your hands. Give it a try; you will see what I am talking about.

Key points:

Volunteering is a good way to keep mentally active.

Volunteering can fill the void of losing your job.

You can choose what you want to volunteer with and for whom. Do your research.

You can volunteer as much or as little as you would like.

You can take a break or stop when you want to. There are no obligations to go beyond your limitations.

You will make great friends and build up your support network.

YOUR NOTES AND THOUGHTS:

Question & Answers

I thought I would add this section so as to answer the questions that I get asked most. The answers are based on research and on what doctors have told me when I posed the question to them; they are also based on my own experience. I will reiterate I am not a clinician but a person with lived experience, and that is how I will answer these questions.

These are also some of the questions I wish I had known the answers to when caring for my mom.

Why do people living with dementia get tired much quicker and sleep more?

There are a number of factors that contribute to this.

As we have discussed, the brain controls every part of your body. The brain uses energy to process information or actions. The more information or actions requested by your body, the more brain power and energy it takes. This is true for all of us and why we all can get mentally tired at times.

The brain is also a very smart organ. This means that as the brain decreases in size, the normal route for processing information or actions may not be available anymore. The brain has the ability to find another route, but that takes brain power.

The problem for a person living with dementia is that the amount of brain power required is much greater than the norm for even day-to-day things. Things you may do without a thought, I will struggle with. The more information or activity required, the more energy used to process it, especially when it comes to processing more than one thing at a time. For example, being part of a group conversation or carrying out multiple tasks consecutively can be challenging.

It was explained to me using this illustration:

Imagine 2 people. Person 1 is healthy, and person 2 is living with dementia. Each has £10 at the start of the day.

They both undertake the same 5 activities during the day. To perform these activities, person 1 will pay £1 for each activity, person 2 will pay £2.

This means person 1 will have £5 afterwards and may choose to do further activities as a result. Person 2, though will have spent all of their money in performing the same activities and cannot do any more.

(In case you haven't figured it out, the money represents the brain power and energy that we have at the start of the day, and the cost is the amount of brain power and energy used to perform the activity.)

When you sleep, your brain tops back up to £10, and you start the next day with the full amount again.

For the person living with dementia, person 2, the more the dementia advances, the more activities will cost. They will also have more broken sleep.

This means that they will run out of brain power much more quickly as time goes on, even when performing the

117

simplest of activities. At this point, the person will need to sleep as they are mentally drained and can no longer function properly.

The brain is also not able to top back up to the full amount due to the broken sleep, and so, as the dementia progresses, they start each day on less and less until the time when they start each day with a deficit. At this point, normally late stage, the person sleeps all the time.

Based on my mom and what I have seen with others, I know that, sadly, at this point, there is not much time left.

Clear as mud? I thought so.

As a carer, I am so tired, what can I do?

Speaking from experience, caring for someone living with dementia is exceptionally tiring and demanding, especially as the dementia progresses.

As we have more broken sleep and perhaps start to wake and move around during the night, it becomes harder to recover from the last day's activities. Sleep is vital for you in order to care for us. You must care for yourself first and foremost.

There are things you can do to help get the sleep you need and to get the breaks you might need (and should take).

The first piece of advice I will give is not to try and keep the person awake through the day if they need to sleep, believing that they will sleep better at night as a result. That only works for a healthy brain. As I explained in the previous question, it is not a matter of choice for me; I need to stop and rest and, if need be, sleep so that I can try and manage the rest of the day. If you want an aggressive and agitated person, try keeping me awake or active!

Keeping the person awake through the day will make no difference to the night activity. What happens is, or what seems to happen to me and what I noticed in my mom, is that we will go into a rapid deep sleep for a length of time and then wake up. I find then once I am awake, I have slept enough. The problem is that it may have only been an hour, which means my wife may only sleep an hour. And so, the problem continues.

Note: If, for some reason, you do need to wake the person up, do so gently. As I have said, the chances are we are in a deep sleep and waking anyone up from that will startle them. I found with myself that if I am woken up harshly, like a nudge on the shoulder and told to wake up, I will have your head. I also find that I am not able to function properly then. It takes me a long while to get back to being 'me'. So, wake them up slowly, gently and with a soft voice. I would also suggest doing so facing the person, but not so close that you are in their face. Remember, peripheral perception may not be working correctly, and we do not want them to think that you mean harm, as it may take a few seconds for them to realise who you are. You do not want a fist in the mouth!

Back to you, as the carer. What can you do?

A number of things are open to you. If the person is like me and can be left alone for an hour or so, take that time to rest and sleep or pop out for a bit. Make sure the person knows that you have your mobile with you and understands how to contact you.

If the person cannot stay alone or it has reached the stage that they cannot use the phone to contact you, then there are alternatives.

Leaving them alone at this stage will result in anxiety and possible wandering. That's the last thing we want.

Speak to your social worker. It is possible to get a person to sit with your loved one for an hour or so. This can be a carer or a PA (personal assistant), which can be a trusted friend should you choose, who is prepared to do this. They can get paid for their time.

Both of the options carry a cost. Some councils will offer a grant to help with the payment of this. If you do not ask, you do not get it. (Grants do not have to be paid back.)

You could just ask a friend who is willing to do this for you voluntarily (which you could sort out yourself).

I chose the PA route. I have a friend that I have known for a long time who is able to take me out a couple of times a week, and for his time I pay him from a grant that we got.

This helps my wife get on with her work and also take the time as she needs for herself.

The other alternative, and this will become more relevant as time passes, is that of respite. This can come in the form of overnight stays or day centres for a few hours. These are charity-based normally and, again, carry a cost.

If you need a good night's sleep or you need a day for yourself then this is a good option (based on your budget).

Note: This is not being selfish, and you are not neglecting your duties as a family member either. It is a necessity to care for yourself first. If you get tired and anxious and it becomes visible to the person with dementia, then they will become anxious and possibly aggressive. The aggression, as we will see later on, can just be because they feel they are the cause of your stress and have no other way of dealing with the problem at hand. Care for yourself!

The other option is one we discussed earlier. The one that takes a lot of thought is that of a care home.

The last thing the person living with dementia, your loved one, would want is for you to put yourself in danger of health concerns or a breakdown as a result of caring for them. I certainly do not want that for my wife or son.

Putting the person in a care home might be the most loving thing you can do. The most guilt-ridden as well, but we will not go there. It will be loving for them so that they can get specialised care but also for you and your health.

Also, remember that a care home means that you will be sleeping apart if it is your wife, husband, or partner, but you can go there every day and spend as long as you like with your loved one. So, it is not the end of the relationship, you are not abandoning them.

Why we feel guilty about getting specialised care for our much-loved family member, I do not know or understand, but we do.

Whatever option you choose, think not only about the person with dementia but also about yourself and what you need. "To care for me, you need to be at your best," is what I tell my wife regularly.

Do not wait for the crisis stage when you are close to burnout. This is not good for you.

As a family, we have discussed this already, while I can. I have instructed my wife and son exactly what to do and when. My future is in my hands, for them to execute so that everyone is cared for.

Can you feel the decline when you have dementia, and what does it feel like?

When asked this question, I often say, "yes, and it's great, I recommend it." I am joking, needless to say. It gets a laugh.

The short answer is yes, at least I do, and I know others have said the same.

At first, you feel something is not quite right; you don't seem to be able to function like you used to. That feeling gets worse as time goes on.

Getting a diagnosis does not change that feeling; it just answers why things are getting worse.

Before, you could do things without even thinking about it, like reading, speaking, being part of a conversation, walking upstairs, picking up a cup or identifying a spoon. Normal day-to-day things become challenging over time. The younger you are when the symptoms start, the harder they are to deal with and mask.

You notice that these things are becoming harder, which, of course, leads to frustration, anxiety, and possibly depression.

In some cases, I liken it to an out-of-body experience; you can feel yourself struggling with a task, for example, but feel powerless to do anything about it. A very strange feeling.

I will also feel the brain getting more and more tired until the point that it hurts to move a finger. I am that mentally drained. The strange thing about it is sometimes I feel I have not done anything during the day to warrant that amount of mental tiredness. But that's how I feel, and there's nothing I can do about it.

I find the weather harder to deal with now, and I find it plays a big role in making my symptoms worse. I suppose when you think about it, we all struggle with tiredness and irritability if the weather is poor for a period of time, such as those rainy and cold days. Amplify that feeling by 10 for someone living with dementia, and you will get an idea of what it is like for us. Care homes will tell you that these days are the days they have the most aggression from residents.

Also, the sun downing effect. Night means sleep, but it is only just past 3 pm. Sunny nights mean staying awake, and early sunrises mean time to get up, even though it is 4 am. This affects the sleep pattern.

The concept of time and the day or year mean nothing to me anymore.

I notice all of these things more now and feel them getting worse.

There is some consolation, though. As the dementia progressed, I noticed for my mom that these feelings started to go away. I think this is due to the brain not being able to comprehend any more what is happening.

For me, now, I manage what I can, I control what I can, and the rest I let go of so as to keep the anxiety down.

You can get medical advice on dealing with these feelings, and there is nothing wrong with accepting medication, either. Just be aware that some of these meds you cannot take with dementia as they will make your symptoms worse. Speak to your doctor or mental health team about this.

Dealing with the symptoms and living with dementia is hard; it takes everything you have to cope. Get the help you need to cope as you need it.

Why do a person's memories regress?

There are a few illustrations you can use here to explain.

I would like you to imagine trying to take items from a large chest and place them all into a shoe box; you'd find it impossible. The same is true for your brain. As the brain shrinks and the hippocampus (the place where memories are stored in the brain) gets smaller or damaged, the less memories it can hold.

Science has taught us that the 'last in, first out' scenario is adopted by the brain, which is why short-term memories are affected first. What I did an hour or day ago, rather than what I did last week or last year.

But you may see that some things seem to stick and can be remembered, whereas others do not. I used that experience in my opening scenario. It's true, this does happen.

I would like you to think about a string of fairy lights. You may know them as Christmas lights.

There are loads of lights on a string. Each light represents a memory.

When the bulb reaches the end of its life, or the string gets damaged, what happens? Normally, a light will stop working if damaged, or if the bulb is going it will flash for a while and then eventually stop altogether.

That is what happens in the brain. If it is damaged, then chances are, those memories are gone and may never be recalled. Head trauma, for example, could cause this, as well as late-stage dementia.

If, however, the brain is shrinking, then it may work sometimes but not others as the neurons fire or misfire. In much the same way as the fairy light flashes for a while, the memory may stick for a while, or it may not. Either way, eventually, the light stops working, and so does the ability to retain that memory.

Why 'first in, last out'?

From the day you are born your brain adds memories – thousands each year, things that have happened that year. I am 50 at the time of writing this, so I have millions of memories stored from each of those years. My 50th year is my last year so far.

Over time, I start to lose memories for the year. The brain works on the concept of last-in, first-out scenario.

For example, over time, I will not remember the 50th year, but I can remember the 49th year. But then 49th year memories start to fall, and I now can only remember from the 48th year down. Then they fall, and so it goes on.

It is said that many seem to be in their mid to late 20s by the time dementia takes their life. What evidence is this based on?

If you have had dealings with a person in late-stage dementia, then you will know based on what they speak about or what memories they have. My mom, for example, could not recognise my dad as, in her mind, he is younger, and she thought I was a baby. I was born when she was 20. She was unable to recollect my brother or sister, even if shown a photograph of them.

If you want to know what age they are in their head, then play some music. The period they respond to identifies their memory year and what memories they hold dear to them. It is a good way to communicate or to start a conversation. Try photos as well and see where they remember.

This is something care homes and care staff forget when dealing with specifically males. Sexual harassment claims are made often by female staff, and the person gets labelled as a perverted old man.

This is not true, and it often comes down to how they treat that man.

Think about it: as a carer, you tell the man, who perhaps in his head is in his 20s or 30s, and you say to him, "let's get you to bed." You take him by the hand and lead him to his bed, where you start undressing him. What is the man supposed to think who, by the way, is still able to be sexually active?

Just putting that out there to help you understand that a person's memory regression is an important thing for you to understand. Knowing what memory age that person is also helps you to understand certain of their behaviours.

Keep in mind also the type of dementia the person has as it is possible that normally the person would know what is right or wrong, but because his filter has been damaged or has gone completely, then what they are doing seems right to them but not to you.

Why do people living with dementia wander?

What we have just answered regarding why memories regress helps to answer this question.

Wandering is often said to relate to anxiety. This is true. But why?

The house that they are in may not be recognisable to the person at that time. Was this the house they grew up in? Have they recently moved? Where does this person think they are or want to be?

Finding the answers to these questions will help you understand why they wander.

If they are not in the home that they are thinking about, then the chances are they want to go home, wherever that may be for them.

Sadly, there is not much you can do about wandering other than putting things in place to stop them from getting out of the house. They should never, however, be locked alone in a house - this is a fire risk.

Put things on the doors to sound an alarm, or that will alert your phone should the door open. There are motion sensors or mats available as well - your occupational therapist can help you with these. I am not a fan of cameras unless this is your partner, wife, or husband, for obvious reasons. Motion detectors, in my opinion, are better.

Trackers are also excellent. Some new technologies enable you to put trackers in their clothing. I know it feels like a spy game, but we want them to be safe at all times and, just in case they do get out, they can be found quickly.

Wandering may not always be wandering outside. It can be that we wander because we cannot remember what we were going to do. I find that. I may wander to the bathroom, then the kitchen or bedroom, because I know there is something I wanted to do but cannot remember what it is.

The worst thing you can do is to shout at the person and tell them to sit down because they are irritating you. You will get a very bad response and it will result in a breakdown of communication and trust. I am not a child.

My wife will gently take me by the hand, standing in front of me, and ask me what I am looking for? If I cannot remember, she will gently lead me to my seat. She will check if I need the loo... we do not want a mess. Though that is to come.

The key is to be gentle and softly spoken at this point. My wife says that I appear glazed at such times. In theory, my brain has shutdown. In old computer terms, it is hanging. Remember those days, ha ha.

Also, a point to remember: never approach from the side or back. This could make the person very stressed and more likely to lash out either in word or action.

All you can do when it comes to wandering, is to gently reassure the person that you are here for them and try your best to restrict their movements outside. But remember, never lock them in a room that is cruel and dangerous, and never leave them in the home alone.

Should I lie to a person living with dementia?

The catch-22 question.

My thoughts on the matter are...

Lying or averting the truth is not uncommon.

We may choose to lie to our children, for example, when it comes to the existence of Santa and what he does. We have, over time even built a whole story relating to him and his reindeer and elves.

We also accept, as we get older, that our parents have lied to us or averted the truth about things in the home or with family to protect us from harm so that we don't worry about things.

We may misdirect the truth from time to time to get ourselves out of a pickle. An example that jumps to my head for some reason might be something like, we went to go and buy a gift that we did not want the person to know about, but when that person asks, "what you were doing today?" you may misdirect and say that you went to the shops to buy something, I don't know, some underwear for yourself. It may well be the truth; perhaps we did, but we neglect to mention what else we bought. We misdirect.

Someone is ill or hurt, we will tell them it will be ok, even when we know it might not be.

So why the concern that we will be lying to the person with dementia?

We believe it is cruel, and we do not want to lie to our loved ones.

That is very true, and we are taught that lying is wrong. But remember what was said in the opening paragraphs of this question: we may choose to do it anyway!

Because the person is confused about memories, where they are and who people are, they will ask questions we will find difficult to answer.

We know the answer, but the truth may cause them to become anxious, irritable, and emotional. We do not want that. The fact that they are asking the question already shows that they are anxious.

If you do not want to lie, find a way to misdirect or give a partial truth. "Will my son be coming to see me tomorrow?" The truth might be no, they are coming up next month because they live far away. Your reply could be perhaps, "he is coming soon".

They will most likely ask the same question again later on. This is not because they do not believe you or they are trying to catch you out thinking that you are lying to them. It is simply because they do not remember.

Therein is the key, in late-stage dementia, when this becomes more relevant, they will not remember your reply. Why say the absolute truth when it is going to cause stress when you could keep them calm with a misdirect or half-truth?

They may make statements that are untrue, misleading or relate to what happened years ago, but they say happened yesterday.

Unless it is absolutely imperative at that time that they need to know the truth, which, let's face it, at this stage will not matter, then ask yourself, "does it really matter that they have mixed things up?"

If the answer is no, then leave it. It does not matter. The last thing you want is an argument or to confuse them more. The person will become withdrawn and see you as the one who always argues with or corrects them. I am sure that is not what you want to be tagged with.

The truth about the matter is this: in my opinion, whatever keeps them calm and stress-free works. It will relieve your anxiety as well by keeping the home peaceful. It will certainly help the care staff as well because they don't want to have to pick up the pieces after you have left them in an agitated state.

No-one wins by being brutally honest all the time. The same is true if we outright lie.

How much you water down the truth, well, that is up to you and your conscience.

For me, I just wanted to see my mom calm. I would hope my loved ones will do the same for me when I am in the same boat.

It really is a matter of what works as long as it keeps the stress levels down for them and for you, and frankly, that may not be the truth.

Why does the person's behaviour change, and how can I handle that?

The simple answer is as the brain changes it affects the way it works.

My mom was a lovely, placid lady. Sure, she could lose her temper, but who doesn't from time to time? She was never known for her temper, though. In fact, very few people even saw her get angry. She was known for her kindness and willingness to help where she could.

As the dementia advanced, we gradually saw her change. She became aggressive and abusive and started using foul language, which she had never done previously. She became a totally different person.

Some of this was a result of frustration as the dementia progressed and her being powerless to change things. I understand this more now that I am living with it; I didn't at the time of caring for her.

Most of it, though, is down to the brain shrinking and no longer working correctly. It's all to do with the frontal part of the brain, where the filter is and where right and wrong are processed.

The person we knew is still in there; after all, it is the same brain. Her inability to recall memories that helped shape her, her brain struggling to filter right from wrong, her inability to speak or express herself, to name just a few things, all contribute to that person's behaviour, possibly changing them into someone we don't recognise.

Irrespective, that person is still your family member and should be treated that way, being shown respect at all times. Retaliation, though hard not to do, should never be an option.

Foul language, for example, is something I am starting to use more often. Unless I hit my finger with a hammer, I would never swear. What has changed?

The brain is complex. The ability to filter right from wrong is something the brain is taught to do from a very young age. Like treating people fairly, not being abusive or judging people, being racist or sexist. These things the brain stores in a box labelled 'do not use', so to speak.

But when the brain starts to struggle with recalling information from the box labelled 'use all the time', and when those neurons do not fire correctly, then the brain looks for another way. It sees a box that has words in them, actions in them, and thoughts in them and thinks I will use that, ignoring the label on the box that says, 'do not use'.

Unfortunately for everyone else, this is generally unacceptable behaviour. It's what clinicians and care home staff will call challenging behaviour.

The problem for the person living with dementia is that to them, there is nothing wrong with what they are doing. Their brain can no longer see that this is the box marked 'do not use'. To them, this is perfectly acceptable behaviour.

How can you deal with it?

"I will show them that this is not acceptable behaviour. I will show them".

That may work for children who are still learning, but it will not work for adults with dementia. Try it and see where it gets you. You can tell me how you got the black eye later on.

If the person is violent, then certainly remove them from the situation. If they are verbally abusive, can you ignore them? Can you overlook the foul language, the sexual remarks, or the dirty joke?

No matter what you do, you will never stop this from happening. You can, however, sometimes control when it happens or even what happens next. Try to understand why it is happening and what is causing the outburst. Often, it is a misunderstanding or the inability to express what they want or need.

Defuse the situation with kindness. I acknowledge that this is not always easy to do, as tempers can flare up, but it must be done if you want to calm the person down.

If you can overlook the situation then that is great.

Do not encourage the language or jokes, no matter how true or funny. By laughing, you encourage them, and because they do not get that much attention anymore, that kind of behaviour becomes a mechanism for attention. Overlook it as much as you can and laugh your head off inside if you wish.

Be firm but gentle and kind at the same time. They will not remember the reprimand, so there is no point in giving it.

Show love right to the end, no matter how bad or embarrassing it may get. That is what you would want; it is what I want, too.

Show empathy. The definition of empathy is to put yourself in their shoes. Picture all that I have just said and what you would want if this was happening to you. Treat the person that way.

One thing to note is that this stage does not normally happen for long before they lose the ability to have bad behaviour, you just need to get through it. Have courage and show love in the meantime.

Conclusion

Get a diagnosis!

As we have seen, there are more advantages to having a diagnosis than there is in wondering what is wrong with you or your loved one.

Yes, at present, the diagnosis process is hard to go through, and there is a lot of stigma you will have to endure, but do not let that put you off. Turn that negative into a positive by using your apprehension, the diagnostic process, and your experience as a training opportunity, a chance to overturn the stigma, one person at a time, if need be.

The key to living with dementia is acceptance by you as the person living with it and by those all-important family members. Be willing to accept support to do this, as it's not easy to do. It will take time and there will be many emotional moments for everyone.

No matter what you decide is best for you and your loved ones, make decisions together and as early as possible while you still can.

Consider the disease and what type of dementia you have, and plan for what the future will look like, but very importantly, always keep one foot in the present!

You do not need to go through this alone. Build up that very important network of people and charities that can support you. There is no need to be afraid of asking for assistance; people will not think less of you. In fact, they admire the courage it takes to do so. Ask, and if need be, insist on the support, especially if it is medically necessary.

By accepting the disease, you will be able to adjust and adapt as needed rather than waiting for it to reach a 'crisis stage'. It will also become easier to recognise when you need to make these changes and do so without it affecting you too much emotionally.

We cannot beat this disease... yet. Many will use the term "living well with dementia." I do not agree with that term. I was living well before I got dementia, but we can live with it to the best of our ability until the time we cannot.

Whatever you decide to do with your days after your diagnosis, the most important advice I could give as a person living with dementia is to make the best use of your time now, live and enjoy life.

Try your hardest not to live in the past. Certainly, think about the past, as there will be very many happy memories there, but try not to think too much about what you could do and now cannot do or struggle with.

Think about how you can adapt to make life easier now. Remember, negative thoughts will get you down, and this can worsen the dementia symptoms and even, in some cases, cause the dementia to move at a more rapid pace. Use your support network if you feel this is happening, and if need be, make use of medication.

Try not to live in the future, either. Plan, get your things in order, and make your wishes known. Living in the future can be just as detrimental to your happiness as living in the past. Plan early - I would say the sooner, the better, and then enjoy the present with peace of mind.

Live in the present as much as you can, enjoy your loved ones, enjoy your time. Do what matters to you while you can. We had all sorts of plans for when we retired. We looked at what was important to us both, and those are the things we have moved forward with. We have prioritised what we can and want to do while I can still enjoy the experience; this has included holidays abroad. We will see how far we get.

Keep your mind and body active, as active as possible. Pick a hobby. I chose gardening. Whatever works for you.

Know your limits, though, and rest as much as you need. When it becomes a frustration rather than fun, then perhaps change the hobby or adapt.

Volunteer. It will certainly keep your mind active, and your experience will be invaluable to those charities you volunteer with. Remember, you can volunteer in whatever role suits you or you feel comfortable with. You can volunteer as much or as little as you like and stop at any time. I highly recommend it, especially if you are looking for that 'work outlet' or want to give something back. Give it a try.

An added advantage are the great friends you will make along the way.

Be that person who supports your mother, father, brother, sister, grandmother, grandfather, or child to the best of your ability. It will not be easy. It will be challenging and, at times, emotionally and physically draining. It is the hardest disease to live with and to care for.

Accept help. There is no need to be a martyr. That is certainly not what I would want for my family.

Take time for yourself – this is very important! It is not being selfish; it is quite the opposite. If you are in a good space, then you can care better.

I cannot stress enough that you must get the support you will need, either now or in the future. The longer you put that off, the worse things will get. I have seen many a carer who has ended up in hospital as a result of mental, emotional, or physical exhaustion because they did not accept or seek out support. Don't let that happen to you!

There is one thing that keeps me going, that keeps me in the fight. A world without dementia. I know it seems farfetched at this point in time, but I am very confident that this will happen. Perhaps not in my lifetime, but it will happen.

Until such a time, fight. Challenge stigma. Challenge and be a part of research!

Enjoy your life. Make a difference. Be the best carer you can.

Remember, there are always people in your corner to help you. You just have to let them help.

I hope these words reassure you that we can live with dementia, that dementia does not spell the end, and that unless you choose to be, you are never alone!

YOUR NOTES, THOUGHTS, AND ACTION PLAN MOVING FORWARD:

Acknowledgements

I would like to take this time to offer a much-needed thank you to some very deserving people. People who have become very close friends and offer support to me on my journey, even when I did not think I needed it.

First and foremost, to my lovely wife and best friend, Aline. I would be lost without you. You have seen the best and the worst of me and have stuck with me through it all, the highs and the lows. I am in awe of the courage you show despite all the challenges we are going through; you face them all with such valour and bravery, I admire that so much in you. When I am having those bad days, you try your best for me to put on that brave face and smile, to try your best to be the support I need, but I know deep inside you are hurting, and sometimes I hear the sobs from the bedroom. I wish I could take the heartbreak and tears away. I feel powerless to make the changes you desperately want, to see me as I was. Knowing that it will get worse over time only hurts more. I will always try to be the support you need, and I will always love you right to the bitter end. Not because you what you do for me but because you said "yes" to becoming my wife, best friend, and my rock. I love you so very much!

Joshua, my beautiful son. Thank you for all that you do for mom and me. For being there for me at all times. Your support and love means the world to us both. I know it is not easy and can be hard to endure, and I certainly do not make it easy some of the time, but I cannot thank you enough for being there in the good times and the bad times. I love you both very much. Son, I am so very proud of the man you have become. With you and the addition of our beautiful daughter-in-law, I know Mom will be in good hands when I can no longer be there for her. We love you son.

Dad, I know this has been hard for you, first with Mom and now with me. You have done the best you could when it came to loving and caring for Mom. I know she would be happy with all that you have done for her. The love you showed her right to the end is an example to us all. I know when you see mom again, she will tell you this. I certainly aspire to be like you and show Aline the same love you showed to Mom despite the challenges you both faced in your time together. Thank you. We know how much you sacrificed to care for Mom right to the bitter end, and it was plain to see by everyone just how much that has taken out of you. Thank you for being there for me as well. You being by my side means the world to me. I love you.

Thank you also to Aline's parents, Gerard and Martine. Despite living in South Africa, they give the best support they can, especially to Aline. They also helped fund the book, to which I will be eternally grateful for, and for their lovely daughter, needless to say.

Alzheimer's Society. Thank you for all the support you have given me and for allowing me to be a part of the family as a volunteer. I know I can be a pain sometimes and be a little forward but sometimes it is the only way to break the mould we find ourselves in. I would specifically like to thank Anna and her great team (I will not name you all in case I forget someone, I would hate to forget someone and have them thinking I do not appreciate them. You all know who you are and have all become good friends, especially you, Anna, taking me under your wing and showing me the ropes). I would also like to thank Kate Lee, Fiona, Caroline, Gemma, Richard, Kate, and Cherie, you are not just colleagues but friends. Keep up the good work. It means a lot to those affected by dementia. Thank you all.

Dementia UK - Young Dementia Network. Thank you for raising the profile of young-onset dementia. I know most of you volunteer your time and resources in addition to your daily jobs which shows just how much you're to see a change being made for young onset. We are in the minority, but you all work so hard to teach people what it is like to live with dementia at a young age; despite this, you are all there fighting against the odds. Thank you.

Bradford University (Clare, Danielle, and the rest of the team). The tireless work you put in for young onset dementia, irrespective of the subtype, cannot be matched. Thank you for your hard work and, for allowing me to be part of your team and for being the first to design an MSC in applied dementia studies. This will be invaluable moving forward in the training of our clinicians and carers. We had a lot of fun in Helsinki. I will always try to remember that. We have the photos.

DEFIN – YD. What a group of ladies! Willing to do anything for any of the volunteers and always smiling. Keep up the good work, and thank you for letting me be a part of the team – Never lose the smile.

Mental Health Team, Hartlepool (Lindsay, Sarah, Gemma, Kath, and all of the PCPG team). Despite being under-resourced and under-manned, you are doing a great job helping so many people with dementia. Thank you for being that support. One of the best in the UK, but you will always be the best in my eyes.

A very BIG special thank you to the Hospital of God (Lawrence, Gail, Nicola, Ian, Rebecca, and the lovely ladies at The Bridge (Hannah, Christine, and Cathrine)) - Our local dementia charity. Thank you for the hard work you put in and for the support you have shown to Aline and myself. Thank you also for the support you show to the Young Onset Dementia Group Hartlepool and for giving us a room to call home. Thank you, also, for the spending of money to convert our cottage, even though I know that this was not easy to do. This will forever be appreciated by myself and Aline. I look forward to finishing the garden and working with you more. Thank you very much from the bottom of my heart.

I would also like to Thank the Young Onset Dementia Group and Lynn. The support you give to us all is invaluable. Providing a safe space to meet with others living with Dementia, providing that all-important support network to us all. Stepping up when so many runaway. Thank you.

Angus, my good friend and PA. Thank you for all the support you give Aline and myself. One day, you may win at ten-pin bowling.

Other charities or organisations that I work with and need to be mentioned and thanked. Alzheimer's Research UK, Brains for Dementia, The Geller Commission, Health Watch

Hartlepool, Dementia Friendly Hartlepool (the odds are against you, yet you keep fighting for those living with dementia in Hartlepool), NIHR and my good friend Michael Curtis.

May all of you mentioned above continue to be that support, not only for me but for all living with or affected by dementia. Continue to be that beacon of light when dementia dims the lights. Dementia needs you. Those living with Dementia and our dearly valued cares need you.

Thank you all for

NEVER ALLOWING US TO BE ALONE!

A special note to past, current, and early career researchers:

Past and current researchers have done so much to get us to the understanding we have of dementia today. You have and are all doing such a great job. We greatly appreciate all that you have done.

Without the research you have done, dementia would be an even dark path to walk. Thank you.

Early career researchers - Dementia needs you!

Your enthusiasm to join the fight against dementia is so greatly appreciated.

Our better understanding of dementia and its causes lies in your hands. Proudly pick up that mantel and continue in the path of past and present researchers.

Thank you for all you do. We appreciate the effort and the time you put in on our behalf. We know you do not have the funding other illnesses have, but despite this, you keep seeking answers, understanding, and treatments.

Remember, a negative outcome to you is still a positive outcome and moves us one step closer to a better understanding.

Keep up the good work!!

Milton Keynes UK
Ingram Content Group UK Ltd.
UKHW050014290824
447448UK00020B/332

9 781917 367240